Orthopaedic Pillow

Shuori Yamada

Orthopaedic Pillow

Theory and Practice

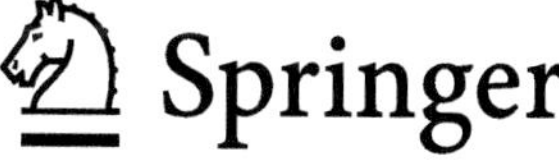

Springer

Shuori Yamada
16 Gou Orthopaedic Clinic
Sagamihara, Kanagawa, Japan

ISBN 978-981-99-0465-5 ISBN 978-981-99-0463-1 (eBook)
https://doi.org/10.1007/978-981-99-0463-1

The translation was done with the help of artificial intelligence (machine translation by the service DeepL.com). A subsequent human revision was done primarily in terms of content.

This Springer imprint is published by the registered company Springer Nature Singapore Pte Ltd.
The registered company address is: 152 Beach Road, #21-01/04 Gateway East, Singapore 189721, Singapore

Preface

Greetings, I am Dr. Shuori Yamada, an orthopedic clinician (pillow evangelist) in Japan. Thank you for your interest in this book.

Pillow, it is a mutual item used for sleep all over the world. However, almost all people, including physicians, do not have correct knowledge about pillows. We have not recognized that pillows are a very important tool to preserve good sleep and health.

My father and I are orthopedic surgeons and have accumulated years of clinical experiences using pillows as a treatment in our clinic. The number of patients we have treated with pillows is over 60,000. The proper use of the pillow as a therapeutic tool has helped many patients with a variety of conditions. I have proven the clinical effects of pillows one by one, and many clinicians have been focusing on these results every year. However, scientific research to show the effects of pillows is still only 16 years old. To be honest, please understand that not everything presented in this book is of a high level of evidence, and that much depends on the author's clinical experiences.

I decided to write this book to help medical professionals and physicians around the world understand what pillow therapy is, an untapped area that has yet to be recognized, to incorporate it into their clinical practice, as well as to promote this new therapy around the world. Adding this pillow therapy to one of your standard treatments is never difficult. Only two are needed, one is the mind of challenging your new treatments and the other is the enthusiasm to wish to improve the patient's symptoms in front of you.

In 2020 the whole world was suffering from an unprecedented COVID-19. In this very COVID-19 disaster, I continued to write this book every day. I am not a respiratory physician or an infectious disease specialist but an orthopedic surgeon unable to treat corona patients on the front lines. That's why I believe how I could contribute to people all over the world from the perspective of my specialty, sleep posture. The answer was to inform clinicians around the world about better sleep and sleep attitudes to develop basic physical fitness that can prevent and treat this infectious disease. So I embarked on the writing of this book. My father and I have developed an algorithm for pillow adjustment based on our experiences in accommodating the pillows of about 120,000 people, including both patients and healthy individuals, since 1972. We strongly hope to use this technology to create a social infrastructure that can remotely monitor optimal sleeping posture so that anyone can sleep peacefully and correctly anywhere in the world. I believe that it is never impossible in a modern community where acceleratedly develop the Big Data Analysis and the Artificial Intelligence.

Sagamihara, Kanagawa, Japan
April 4, 2022

Shuori Yamada

Acknowledgments

I pay tribute to my late father, Dr. Hidemaru Kumagai, who discovered the world's only original treatment, "Pillow Therapy," 50 years ago and gave her the opportunity to inherit it. I am also grateful to Dr. Toru Suguro who supported me in challenging this grand subject 20 years ago. I am sincerely grateful to Dr. Daisuke Kurosawa for giving me this rare opportunity to compile my life's work into this book. I am grateful to Professors Ko Matsudaira and Hiroyuki Oka for teaching me the design and practical guidance of this five-year multicenter study and also to Professor Tohru Hoshi for his expertise and help in data analysis and statistical analysis. I am grateful to Dr. Yasuhisa Tanaka, a leading expert in cervical spine research, for his interpretive advice on our results. We thank Dr. Michio Toda and Physiological Therapist Takahiro Tsuge, who believe most deeply in the theory and effects of the pillow and engage in productive discussions. I deeply appreciate Kokoro Yamada for leading the challenging survey of people in the U.S. and other countries around the world using the Internet. Finally, I sincerely thank Mr. Kenichiro Tsumura for his invaluable advice in English editing.

About This Book

To date, there is a paucity of studies and publications on clinical treatment using pillows, and in addition, few clinicians are interested in such treatment.

First of all, it is important to be aware of the effectiveness of pillow therapy and to be interested in it. Chapter 1 introduces them to you.

In Chap. 2, we present the definition and positioning of pillow therapy and the relationship between pillows and treatments. If researchers and clinicians, especially those outside Japan, can understand our pillow theory and how it differs from your current therapies, new treatment options may open the world.

Chapter 3 specifically introduces the various diseases and conditions for which pillow therapy is effective.

In Chap. 4, I organize the fundamental knowledge of pillow therapy. Clinicians can implement the pillow therapy for their patients in the clinics after reading this chapter.

In Chap. 5, we demonstrated the number of basic and clinical studies on how we have developed our theory of pillow adjustment and evidences supporting our claims. You will be introduced to a new treatment unique in the world.

In Chap. 6, we list various questions we have received from patients and the answers to them during our 20 years of "The Pillow Clinic" as a specialty outpatient clinic. This Q&A will help you to answer questions from your patients when you treat them with pillows in the future. In addition, we provide information on bedding including bed mattresses, comforters, and pajamas that affect sleep posture, as well as the sleep environment in general.

Contents

About the Author

Shuori Yamada, MD, PhD graduated from Tokyo Women's Medical University School of Medicine in 1989. She is an orthopedic surgeon. After working at university hospitals and city hospitals, She became the vice president of Naruse Orthopedic Clinic in 2002 and the director of 16 Gou Orthopedic Clinic in 2007. Her main research field is sleep posture, and in 2003 she founded a venture company, Yamada Shuori Pillow Research Institute, Co., Ltd. and serves as its president. Her major publications are:

Yamada S. Pillow Revolution: Our Body Will Change Overnight. Tokyo: KODANSHA LTD; 2004.

Yamada S, Hoshi T. Sleep Posture Revolution: MAKURA in BED Will Change People's Whole Life. Tokyo: NIPPON HYORON SHA CO., LTD; 2014.

Yamada S. Pain Disappears When Neck Posture Is Changed. Tokyo: FOREST Publishing Co., Ltd.; 2015.

Yamada S. 15 Million People Love to Use the Woolen Cervical Pillow. New Taipei City: ECUS CULTURAL ENTERPRISE LTD; 2015.

Yamada S. The Novel Pillow-Head Health Method. Taichung: Morning Star Publishing Inc.; 2015.

Pillow for Therapy

1

Abstract

Awareness among clinicians regarding treatment with pillows is far from high. However, once the effectiveness of this method is learned, you should be willing to try this method, aided by its safety and simplicity. The aim of this chapter is to motivate you to become aware of, interested in, and willing to utilize in your clinical practice the benefits and safety of "treating by using pillows" for clinicians. Pillows are effective for a variety of orthopedic and other medical conditions. To begin with, we present the results of clinical studies on intractable shoulder stiffness, for which pillows are most effective. My two primary studies presented in this chapter examined not only shoulder stiffness but also other symptoms as well. However, the effects are probably most strongly felt when the pillow is used on patients with intractable stiff shoulders. If you are interested in the effectiveness and safety of the pillow therapy, try it on your patients. We will explain the specific procedures in Chap. 4.

Keywords

Pillow · Pillow therapy · Neck pain · Shoulder stiffness · Clinical research · Somatic Symptom Scale-8 (SSS-8)

Supplementary Information The online version contains supplementary material available at https://doi.org/10.1007/978-981-99-0463-1_1.

S. Yamada, *Orthopaedic Pillow*, https://doi.org/10.1007/978-981-99-0463-1_1

1.1 Introduction

First, let's discuss "treating by using pillows (and their adjustments)" (hereafter referred to as pillow therapy). The levels of knowledge of pillow therapy vary from clinician to clinician. Dr. A, who knows little about pillow therapy, and Dr. B, who has a little knowledge about pillow therapy, may each have the following questions.

Dr. A's questions about pillow (in case of persons who hardly know anything about pillow therapy)

- Nowadays, my patients often ask me what type of pillow should be used.
- What pillow shall I recommend to him/her?
- Can I recommend a commercially available contour pillow?

Dr. B's questions about pillow (in case of persons who know a bit about pillow therapy)

- Can I recommend feather, urethane, or buckwheat pillows?
- Why is the contour pillow not good enough?
- What is the correct cervical spine alignment during sleeping?
- Is sleep position affected by both pillow and mattress?
- Is a pillow so good for our health?

I suggest you read first "The Effects of Pillow Therapy on Cervical Pain and Shoulder Stiffness (Sects. 1.2.1 and 1.2.2), " not only if you are interested in the effects of pillows but also if your knowledge is at the level of Dr. A or Dr. B. The reason why you should read this data first is that the results most directly demonstrate the effectiveness and importance of pillow therapy. As you are reading these data, you will be intrigued by the effectiveness of pillow therapy and will want to read more. Then, by the time you have read all of the studies, you will be a Dr. Pillow recommending the pillow therapy (Fig. 1.1). Pillow therapy is thus a simple, effective, and efficient treatment procedure. However, this method has not yet been recognized worldwide. Although it may sound a bit far-fetched and eccentric, I have experienced time and again the power of adjusting the pillow to patient's needs to improve his/her pain and sleep, ultimately energizing both the mind and body. We call this as the five E elements of Pillow Therapy (i.e., first E is Easy; second E is Effective; third E is Efficient; fourth E is Extraordinary; and fifth E is Encourage) (Fig. 1.2).

Pillow therapy does not compete with any other therapies and should serve as the foundation, or infrastructure, for a variety of different therapies. Specifically, when a patient comes to the clinic with a chief complaint of neck pain, currently the clinician may plan a variety of treatments, including medication, injections, rehabilitation, and so on. However, prior to these treatments, the physician should provide sleeping postural guidance, or pillow guidance that is the basis or foundation (i.e., infrastructure) of daily life. This is because if the infrastructure is poor, no matter what treatments are provided on it, they will not suitably work.

Pillow therapy does not require patients to do anything special. It is simply a matter of adjusting patient's currently using pillow, which has not any medical evidence or criteria, based on a certain criterion presented in this book.

Pillow therapy is not a treatment performed solely by a physician. Like many other illnesses, it is a treatment that the medical team should work on, as the nurse's lifestyle guidance and as the physical therapist's postural guidance. When the patient's symptoms improved successfully, the whole team members can realize the benefits of the pillow therapy.

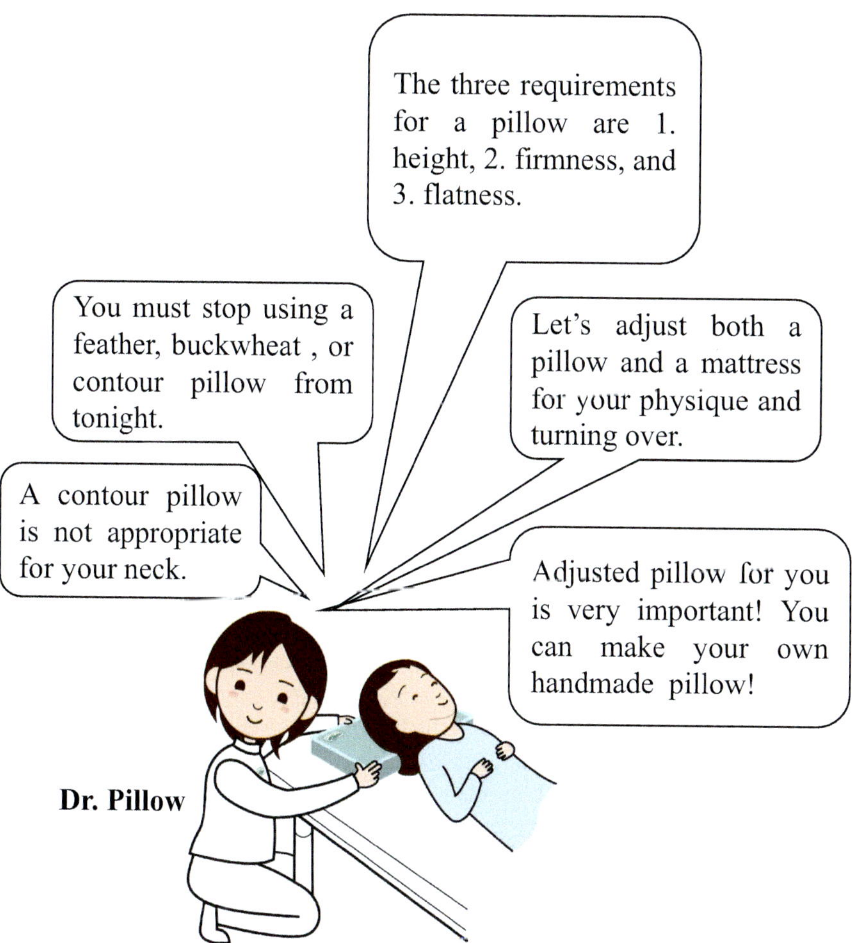

Fig. 1.1 Clinician who specializes in pillow therapy (one who recommends pillow therapy)

Fig. 1.2 Five E elements of an adjusted pillow

1st E: Easy
2nd E: Effective
3rd E: Efficient
4th E: Extraordinary
5th E: Encourage

1.2 Try Pillow Therapy for Intractable Shoulder Stiffness

I have been frequently asked by physicians who are interested in pillow therapy. They uniformly ask as “I’m going to instruct my patients to adjust their pillows, but which cases should I start with first to realize the benefits?” My answer is “First of all, I recommend starting in patients with intractable cervical pain or shoulder stiffness. If the patient has symptomatic ones, it does not matter what the cause is, such as osteoarthritis or a cervical disc herniation. Even in cases not responding well to other conservative therapies, the efficacy can usually be confirmed 2 weeks at the earliest or within 3 months on average.”

Although “neck pain or stiff shoulders” is a very common symptom, patients actually feel a long-term physical burden due to this complaint, which may lead to psychosocial disturbances as well. In Japan, stiff shoulders have always ranked first or second as a complaint of people in the Comprehensive Survey of Living Conditions conducted by the Ministry of Health, Labor and Welfare since 1980. However, no definitive treatment for the symptom has yet been established.

Neck pain is a public health problem for the general population worldwide, but the situation varies from country to country considerably. Improving health data on musculoskeletal conditions such as neck pain in all countries and regions is strongly suggested to improve the global burden of disease [1]. The intensity of chronic pain, such as chronic neck pain, has been reported to be significantly associated with insomnia in chronic pain patients [2]. A vicious cycle may have developed in which sleep disturbance exacerbates pain, and insomnia caused by pain further exacerbates pain. Since around 2010, there have been many reports on the association between insomnia, pain, and depression [3–5], as well as the association between chronic pain in various parts of the body and sleep disorders in diseases of the musculoskeletal system [6, 7]. In a systematic review with a meta-analysis by Thomas Bilterys et al. [8] published in 2021, insomnia was found to be relatively common in people with chronic spinal pain (CSP). They also found that key factors in the association of CSP with insomnia were high pain intensity scores, depressive symptoms, and anxiety. The establishment of new effective treatments for both chronic neck pain and sleep disorders is awaited.

I believe that pillow therapy becomes one of them. It is important for physicians to first experience and realize the safety and effectiveness of pillow therapy and how simple and effective it is. We have seen this simple, noninvasive treatment makes release many patients from long-suffering symptoms and to be happy. It is the greatest joy for our physicians to see a patient smile and say, "I followed your instructions and I feel better." I want as many clinicians as possible to experience this feeling.

Let us specifically demonstrate the effectiveness of the pillow therapy using data of two clinical trials in patients with neck pain and shoulder stiffness.

First, Clinical Study 1 was a retrospective study of the medical records from 2007 to 2013 of patients who have attended our clinic with the main complaints of neck pain and shoulder stiffness. The results of this study showed that the pillow therapy was effective for shoulder stiffness, and we realized that the therapy was also effective for somatic symptoms, so we developed a hypothesis and planned the next study. Next, Clinical Study 2 was titled "Efficacy verification of pillow adjustment for patients with neck pain and shoulder stiffness with somatic symptoms."

1.2.1 Clinical Study 1: A Retrospective Study on Effects of Pillow Adjustment in Patients with Neck Pain and Shoulder Stiffness

1.2.1.1 Purpose

To investigate whether cervical spine alignment management by pillow adjustment during sleep improves neck pain, shoulder stiffness, and accompanying somatic symptoms.

1.2.1.2 Subjects and Methods

This is a retrospective study analyzing medical record data and MRI findings of cervical spine alignment of patients who had presented to our clinic from 2004 to 2013 and underwent pillow adjustments for cervical spine disorders.

Among preliminary selected patients, patients who had taken MRI of the cervical spine and received their pillow adjustment were enrolled for the study.

Patients' main complaints of "shoulder stiffness in the broad sense" and "somatic symptoms" as well as objective findings were evaluated using the number of patients who improved before and after optimal pillow use/number of patients with complaints (improvement ratio, hereafter IRs). Subjective symptoms were scored on a 3-point scale of 2 (strong subjective symptoms), 1 (light subjective symptoms), and

0 (no subjective symptoms), and tests of significance were conducted before and after pillow use. For other subjective findings, tests of significance were conducted between the measurements before and after pillow use.

Subjective symptoms consist of three shoulder stiffnesses [(a) neck and shoulder stiffness; (b) neck pain; and (c) upper limb pain] and three somatic symptoms (d) headache; (e) dizziness; and (f) insomnia]. Objective findings include g) ROM of cervical spine extension, (h) ROM of cervical spine flexion, (i) tenderness score (trigger points score), (j) Spurling test, (k) upper limb muscle strength, and (l) upper limb perception. Improvement in the objective findings is defined as lightness or resolution of the abnormal items.

Data Analysis

The results are shown as improvement ratio (IRs), i.e., number of improved patients at post-pillow adjustment divided by total number of patients with symptom/finding at baseline, mean values of scores or measurements before and after pillow use, and P values. The results of those cases that were not able to test due to insufficient sample-size are shown as "-". The significant level for hypothesis testing was set at $P = 0.05$.

The effects on patients' main complaint of "shoulder stiffness in the broad sense" as well as their somatic symptoms and objective findings were evaluated using each of IRs. Subjective symptom is scored on a 3-point scale of 2 (severe), 1 (mild or moderate), and 0 (negative).

1.2.1.3 Results

A total of 410 patients (195 males and 215 females; 14–93 years old, mean age 50.5) were enrolled in the study. The mean duration of use of the adjusted pillow was 110.9 days.

The IRs and P values for subjective symptoms of shoulder stiffness in the broad sense are as follows: (a) neck and shoulder stiffness, 70.9% (n = 78/110), $P < 0.01$; (b) neck pain, 76.1% (n = 153/201), $P < 0.01$; (c) upper limb pain, 78.6% (n = 66/84), $P < 0.01$; (d) headache, 64.9% (n = 37/57), $P < 0.01$; (e) dizziness, 65.2% (n = 15/23), $P < 0.01$; and (f) insomnia, 76.9% (n = 20/26), $P < 0.01$, and for objective findings: (g) ROM extension, 43.3% (n = 84/194), $P > 0.05$; (h) ROM flexion, 42.8% (n = 80/187), $P < 0.05$; (i) Tenderness score, 63.4% (n = 102/161), $P < 0.01$; (j) Spurling test, 65.4% (n = 17/26), $P < 0.05$; (k) Upper limb muscle strength, 40.0% (n = 2/5), $P > 0.05$; and l) Upper limb perception, 48.6% (n = 17/35), $P > 0.05$. Figure 1.3 shows the number of patients with complaints, the number of improved patients, and IRs (upper figure), and the mean of scores or measurements and the results of significance difference tests, for all subjective symptoms and objective findings.

In subjective symptoms, the percentage of patients with cervical spine disease who reported 3 symptoms (a–c) of shoulder stiffness as their chief complaint at baseline ranged between 84 and 201 out of 410 patients, and the IRs were greater than 70% for all symptoms. The percentage of patients complaining of the three somatic symptoms (d–f) at baseline ranged between 23 and 57 of 410 patients, and

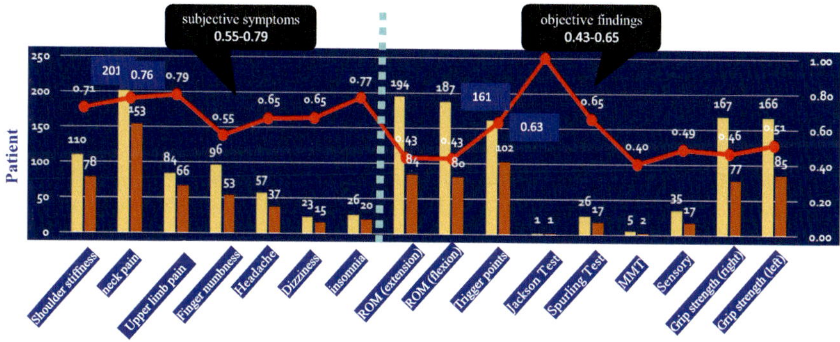

Breakdowns of patients (a bar graph) and IRs (a line graph)

Before use of the optimal pillow (yellow bars)

After use of the optimal pillow (orange bars)

IRs (red solid line, the right Y-axis)

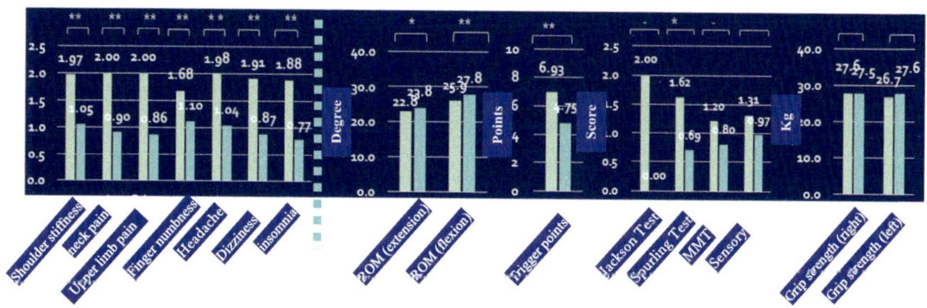

Statistical testing outcoms for symptom improvement

Before use of the optimal pillow (Green bars)

After use of the optimal pillow (Blue bars)

Fig. 1.3 Result 1. Details of improved patients and IRs on subjective symptoms and objective findings

the IRs were minimum of 60% for all symptoms. All three shoulder stiffness symptoms (a–c) and somatic symptoms (d–f) improved statistically significantly after pillow adjustment.

The improvement of objective findings was defined as improvement or disappearance of abnormalities, but only ROM, number of tender points, and Spurling test showed significant improvement.

Conversely, as the improvement in objective findings (g–l) is defined as lightness or resolution of the abnormal items, their IRs were between 40% and 65% with only (h) ROM flexion, (i) Tenderness score, and (j) Spurling test showing statistically significant improvements.

For MRI findings, in 96 patients with cervical disc degeneration, subjective symptoms (a), (b), (c), and (d) were significantly improved. In 194 patients with cervical disc bulging or herniation, subjective symptoms (a) to (d), and objective findings (h), (i), and (j) were significantly improved, and in 58 patients with cervical spinal canal stenosis, subjective symptoms (a) to (c), and objective findings (i) were significantly improved. Figure 1.4 shows details of improvements and IRs on MRI-based symptoms of cervical disc diseases.

The number of patients complaining of the three symptoms (a–c) of stiff shoulders was observed most frequently in patients with cervical disc herniation, in which IRs were as high as 80% or more. Comparing the IRs of the former cervical disc herniation and the latter cervical disc degeneration, the result was shoulder stiffness (82% vs. 35%), neck pain (85% vs. 57%), and upper limb pain (84% vs. 47%). In short, IRs of patients with cervical disc herniation (n = 194), which is considered more severe in general, are higher than patients with cervical disc herniation ($n = 96$) (Fig. 1.4). By age, the three symptoms of shoulder stiffness in subjective symptoms as well as headache and insomnia in somatic symptoms showed a tendency to increase in improvement rates, especially at age 50 and older. Comversely, no age-related trend was observed in objective findings (Fig. 1.5). Symptom improvement rates were 79% (66/84) and 82% (69/84) after 2 weeks and 3 months of pillow

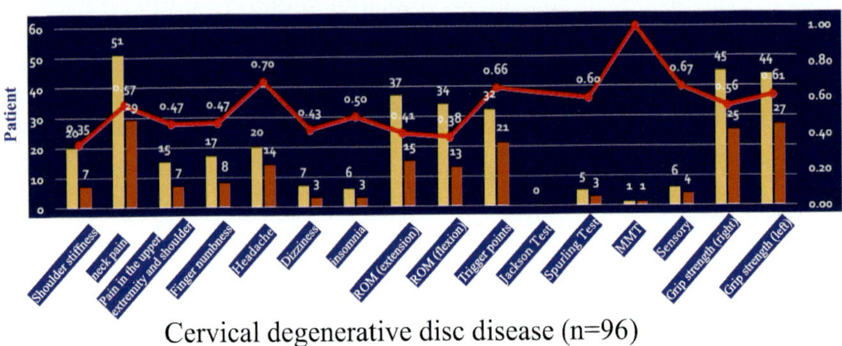

Cervical degenerative disc disease (n=96)

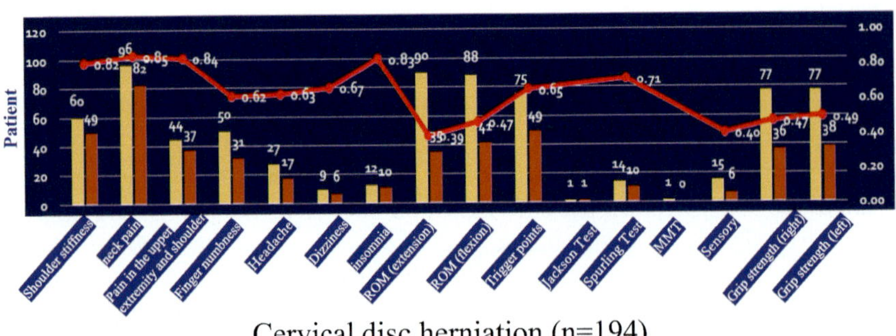

Cervical disc herniation (n=194)

Fig. 1.4 Details of improvements and IRs on MRI-based symptoms of cervical disc disease

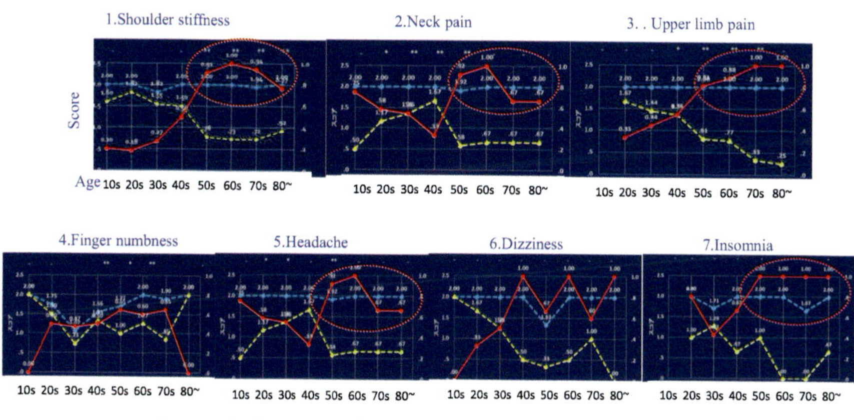

Scores before use of the optimal pillow (blue dotted line)
Scores after use of the optimal pillow (yellow dotted line)
IRs (red solid line, the right Y-axis)

Fig. 1.5 Scores and IRs by age groups—subjective symptoms

therapy, respectively, and satisfaction rates were 83% (70/84) and 83% (70/84) in the same manner (Fig. 1.6).

1.2.1.4 Discussion

In this study, the clinical effects of pillow adjustment were statistically evaluated by classifying shoulder stiffness into three dimensions, i.e., "shoulder stiffness in the broad sense," "somatic symptoms," and objective findings. As a result, stiffness in the broad sense (shoulder stiffness, neck pain, and upper limb pain) and somatic symptoms (headache, dizziness, and insomnia) indicated high IRs between 65% and 79% (see Fig. 1.3 upper).

In cases where psychosocial stress becomes pronounced as physical symptoms, it is called somatization, and the concept of somatization becoming pronounced and leading to functional disorders is called functional somatic syndromes (FSS) [9].

Recently, Japanese orthopedic surgeons believe that intractable shoulder stiffness may be included in a category of FSS. Many of the patients in this study complained of intractable stiff shoulders that interfered with Activities of Daily Living (ADL) for a long term, ranging from several years to more than 30 years, and I also believe that the stiffness falls into the category of FSS. Although the mechanism by which pillow adjustment improves intractable stiff shoulders, a category of FSS, has not yet been determined, this study suggests that adjusting sleep posture can improve somatic symptoms.

As described above, I conducted the retrospective study on shoulder stiffness named Clinical Study 1, which confirmed improvements in most subjective symptoms of shoulder stiffness and in several objective findings. I realized that this

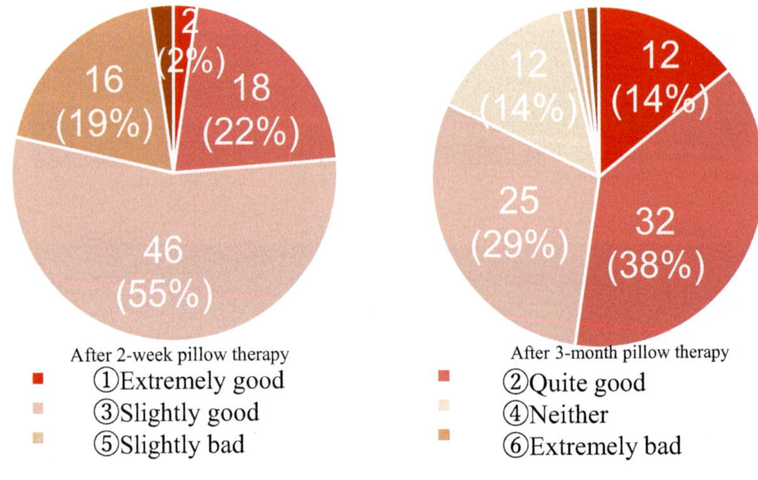

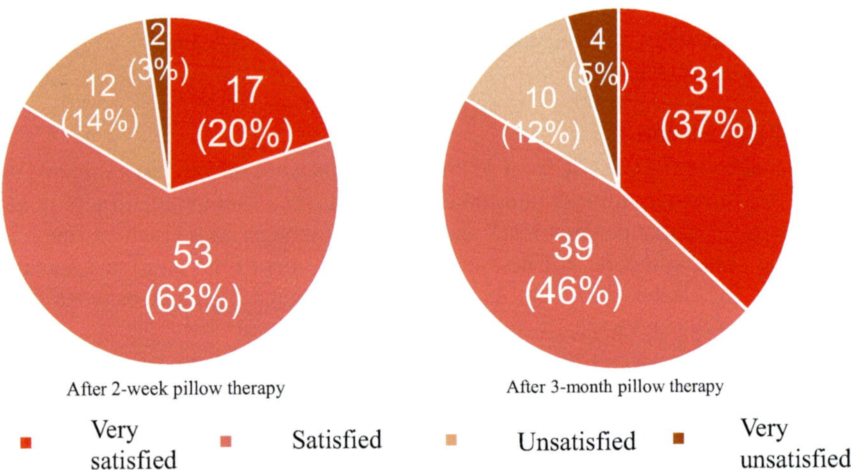

Fig. 1.6 Symptom improvements and treatment satisfaction ($N = 84$)

study confirms what I have always felt the effectiveness of the pillow in my clinical practice. That is the improvement of somatic symptoms (headache, dizziness, insomnia, and so on). Based on the Clinical Study 1 outcomes, we planned a next prospective study. The study was a prospective, multicenter study conducted in three medical institutes including the 16 Gou Orthopedic Clinic, Kurashiki Medical Center, and the Department of Medical Research and Management for Musculoskeletal Pain, twenty-second Century Medical and Research Center, The University of Tokyo.

1.2.2 Clinical Study 2: Effects on Pillow Adjustment for Patients with Shoulder Stiffness and Neck Pain with Somatic Symptoms

1.2.2.1 Background

In recent years, patients with chronic musculoskeletal pain may have frequently sleep disturbances [2, 4, 7, 8]. Insomnia is a common secondary symptom of chronic pain because of the bidirectional relationship between pain and sleep [5].

In a patient with chronic neck pain, his/her sleep disturbances can cause a vicious cycle of increased pain sensitivity, which can further increase the pain. However, there is no treatment strategy yet that simultaneously improves both chronic neck pain and sleep disorder.

1.2.2.2 Purpose

The cause of intractable neck pain and shoulder stiffness may be a combination of physical and psychosocial stresses in the patient.

In cases where psychosocial stress becomes pronounced as physical symptoms, it is called somatic symptoms, including the following eight ones: stomach or bowel problems; back pain; pain in arms, legs, or joints; headache; chest pain or shortness of breath; dizziness; feeling tired or having low energy; and trouble sleeping.

We investigated whether cervical spine alignment management by pillow adjustment during sleep improves neck pain, shoulder stiffness, and accompanying somatic symptoms.

1.2.2.3 Subjects and Methods

Study population: Patients with a score of 8 or higher (moderate or higher) on the Somatic Symptom Scale-8 (SSS-8) [10] who visit the site with a chief complaint of neck pain and shoulder stiffness.

Eligibility criteria: The inclusion criteria were patients who (1) visited the hospital complaining of neck pain or stiff shoulders with or without upper extremity radiating pain, with a score of 8 or higher on the SSS-8 and a score of 2 or higher on the insomnia item, (2) provided written consent; and (3) understood how to adjust the pillow and were able to use it as instructed. The exclusion criteria were patients who (1) wished to receive medication, rehabilitation, or physical therapy at the time of participation in this study; (2) had obvious findings of cervical myelopathy and had indication for surgical treatment, and (3) judged by the investigator in charge to be inappropriate for participation in this study.

Prohibited therapies: No additional medication, rehabilitation, physical therapy, or orthotic therapy was allowed for the subjects after joining the study. If a subject was receiving any other medications as a pre-treatment, the dose and administration must not be change during the study.

The study was interrupted if a subject refused to continue the study (i.e., withdraw his/her informed consent) or if the investigator judged to start concomitant therapy, such as medication, due to degradation of symptoms such as pain.

After the subjects had used the pillow for 2 weeks, they were interviewed about adjusting the height of the pillow. If subject's head did not fall off the pillow upon waking, it was judged that the subject understood how to adjust the pillow and used it properly.

Study procedure: After submitting a consent form, A candidate of subjects completes the SSS-8 self-administered questionnaire to evaluate the degree of somatic symptom burden. The questions of SSS-8 are started with the main instruction "During the past 7 days, how much have you been bothered by any of the following problems?" and followed by eight sub-questions: (1) stomach or bowel problems, (2) back pain, (3) pain in your arms, legs, or joints, (4) headaches, (5) chest pain or shortness of breath, (6) dizziness, (7) feeling tired or having low energy, and (8) trouble sleeping. Each sub-question was rated on a 4-point scale of 0 (not at all), 1 (a little), 2 (somewhat), 3 (a lot), and 4 (very much), and the total score out of 32 (4 × 8) points determined the somatic symptom burden. Then, candidates with the total score of 8 and over (i.e., patients with medium, high, or very high burden) are enrolled in the study.

Subjects were not instructed on how to adjust their posture during the daytime, except when asked.

Study pillow: Subject used various types and materials of pillow before the study. They were provided with a handmade pillow adjusted to the optimal height for individual subject using the "Set-up for Spinal Sleep" Method (SSS Method, Fig. 1.7)

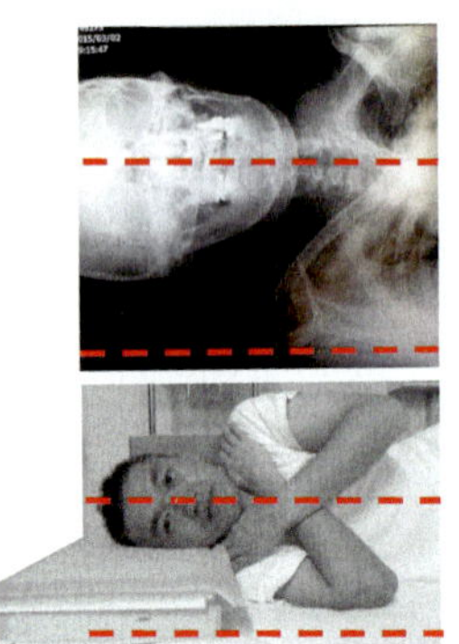

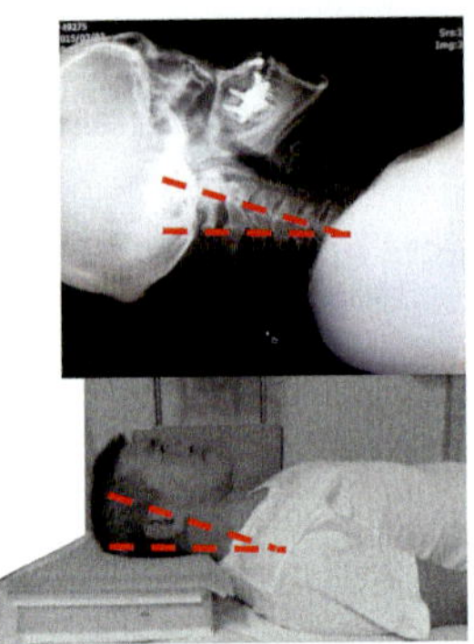

1st step: In the lateral position 2nd step: In the supine position

Set up for Spinal Sleep method (SSS method) is a method adjusting the height of -pillow for each person.

1st step: In the lateral position, the pillow height is adjusted so that the axis of head and trunk of the subject is aligned in parallel with the bed surface.

2nd step: In the supine position, the cervical spine is held at an angle of approximately 15 degrees anterior tilt from the bed surface.

3rd step: In the dynamic motion, we check how smoothly the subject is able to turn over according to the different height of pillow, adjusting increments and decrements of 5mm.

Finally, the pillow height that enables the subject to turn over most smoothly is the optimal adjusted pillow.

Fig. 1.7 Set up for Spinal Sleep Method (SSS Method) (JP2004209099A)

developed by ourselves. The material of handmade pillow was Japanese entrance mat and towelket (a blanket made of toweling) (Fig. 1.8). The details of the SSS Method are explained in Sect. 4.4.

Endpoints: Primary endpoint was changes in SSS-8 total score from baseline to 2 weeks and 3 months after using the adjusted pillows. Secondary endpoints were SSS-8 changes by burden severities, changes in the Numerical Rating Scale (NRS) for the severity of neck pain and shoulder stiffness.

Data analysis: SSS-8 scores and NSRs were summarized in mean ± SD. Comparisons were tested using Wilcoxon's signed rank test and the significant level for hypothesis testing was set at $P = 0.05$.

1.2.2.4 Results

The protocol, informed consent form, and study materials were investigated and approved by the Ethics Committee of Kurashiki Medical Center prior to commencing any study procedures. We acquired the written consent from all subjects using the approved informed consent form before starting the study.

Eighty-four patients out of 95 eligible and with a score of 8 or higher (moderate or higher) on the SSS-8 were included in the study. Subjects were 24 (28.6%) males and 60 (71.4%) females with a mean age of 50.1 years. The mean duration since the onset of the chief complaint was 104 months (8.8 years), and the median was 36 months (3.0 years). A total of 60 (71.4%) subjects had visited other departments including orthopedics, neurosurgery, pain clinic, psychiatry/psychosomatic medicine, and sleep medicine during the period. The type and material of pillows currently used by subjects were also interviewed (Fig. 1.8); the most three were standard pillow (n = 26, 31%), wave pillow (n = 17, 20%), and center dimple or segmented pillows (n = 11, 13% each).

There was no significant difference in baseline characteristics including sex, age, BMI, and smoking habits. Severities of burden load (SSS-8 total score) at baseline were 39 subjects for moderate (score: 8–11), 20 for high (score: 12–15), and 25 for very high (score: 16 and over).

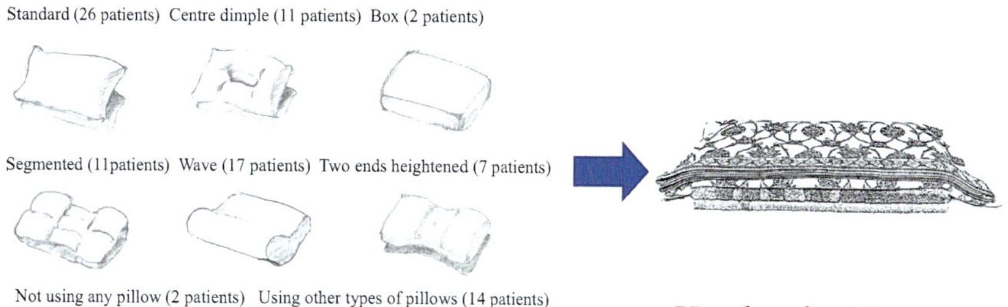

Type and material of pillows used by subjects before the study

Japanese entrance mat and towelket (a blanket made of toweling)

Fig. 1.8 Handmade pillow used in the study

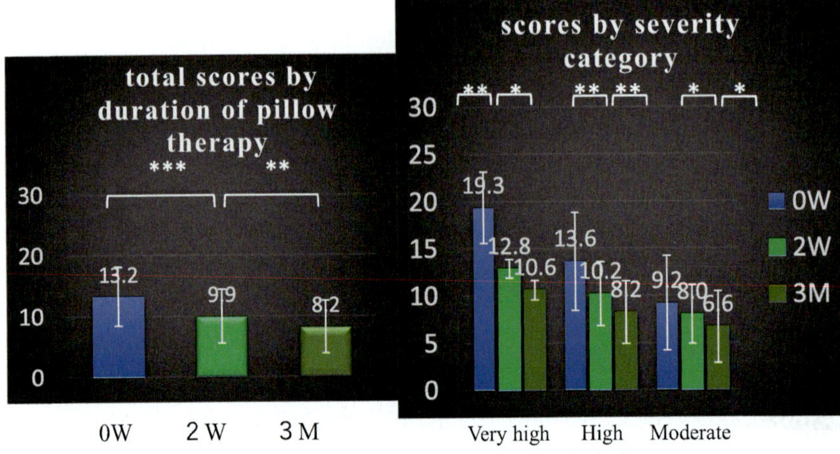

Fig. 1.9 Mean changes of SSS-8 scores in total and by severity ($N = 84$)

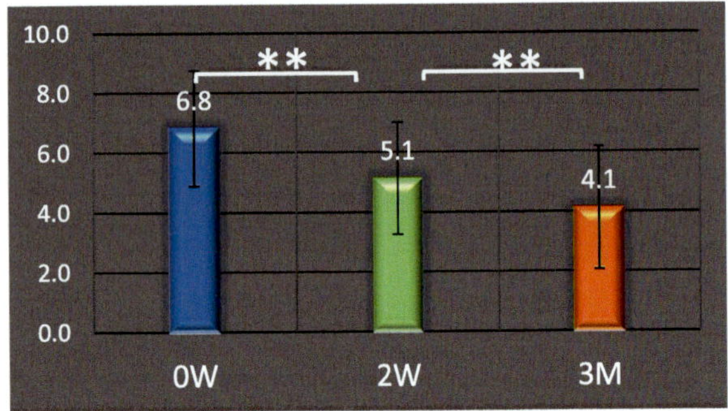

Fig. 1.10 Mean changes of NRS scores by time points ($N = 84$)

The outcomes of primary endpoint, mean changes of SSS-8 total score from baseline to 2 weeks and 3 months after using the adjusted pillows, were −4.0 at 2 weeks and −5.0 at 3 months with statistically significant ($P < 0.001$) each (Fig. 1.9 left).

Mean changes of SSS-8 classified by burden severity, moderate ($n = 39$), high ($n = 20$), and very high ($n = 25$) groups, were −1.0, −3.5, and −6.0 at 2 weeks and −3.0, −5.0, and −7.0 at 3 months with statistically significant ($P < 0.05$) each (Fig. 1.9 right). There was a trend that the higher the baseline SSS-8 severity, the higher the degree of improvement.

Mean changes of NRS for the severity of neck pain and shoulder stiffness were −2.0 at 2 weeks and −3.0 at 3 months with statistically significant ($P < 0.01$) each (Fig. 1.10). Mean score changes of 8 sub-groups (symptoms) of SSS-8 were all

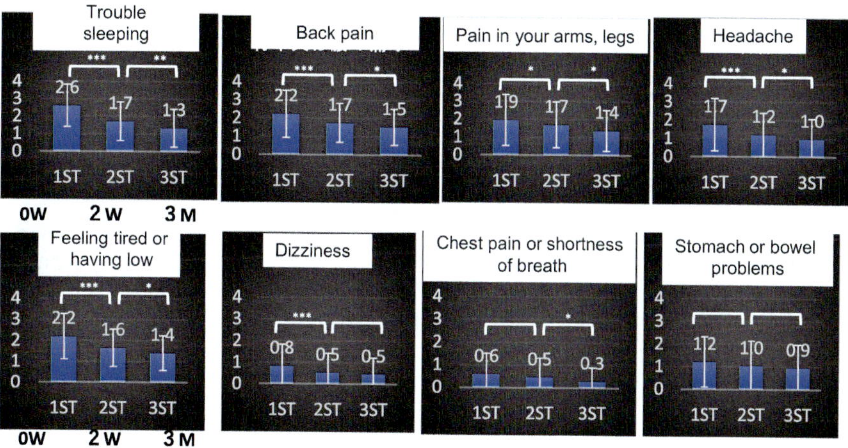

Fig. 1.11 Mean scores of 8 sub-groups (symptoms) in SSS-8

significantly improved ($P < 0.05$), except "Stomach or bowel problems," during the study period (Fig. 1.11). The most significantly improved symptom was "Trouble sleeping" (mean score: 2.6 → 1.3). The overall symptom improvement ratios were 79% (66/84) at 2 weeks and 82% (69/84).

1.2.2.5 Case Reports

Case 1

An 80-year-old woman, height: 150 cm, and body weight: 47.5 kg. Her complications were stroke, dementia, hypertension, atrioventricular block, esophageal hiatal hernia, liver cyst, bronchial asthma, and multiple thoracolumbar compression fractures.

She has cervical pain since 33 years old, but a fall at the age of 65 induced the exacerbation of cervical pain and tension in the cervical muscles. After that, she developed loss of appetite, dizziness, headache, eye pain, ear pain, right shoulder pain, arousal due to pain while sleeping, back pain, lower limb pain, and numbness and cramp of the lower limbs. In the standing posture, she had a severe rounded back and therefore needed a cane or assistance from others to maintain her standing position. In the supine posture, she was not able to lengthen the spine because of her constructed kyphosis due to a compression fracture of the thoracolumbar vertebrae (Fig. 1.12). She came to our hospital after consulting three orthopedic surgeons. The type of pillow she had been using was a pillow with high sides and low center, made of high elastic urethane. Her optimal pillow height we determined was 90 mm, which was very high compared with persons without kyphosis. Sagittal balance was lower in the supine position than in the standing position when comparing the X-ray standing and supine positions (Fig. 1.13). Two weeks after the pillow adjustment, her cervical tightness and right shoulder pain decreased, headache almost disappeared, and therefore she stopped taking medication. Three months later, her SSS-8

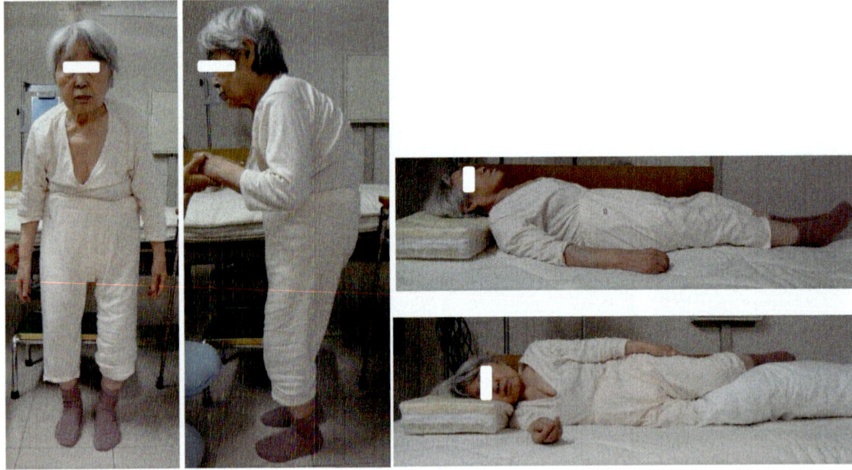

An 80-year-old woman cries with night pain.
Her main complaints are "I can't sleep" and "I vomit when I turn over during sleeping".

Fig. 1.12 Case 1. Standing and recumbent postures in a patient with kyphosis

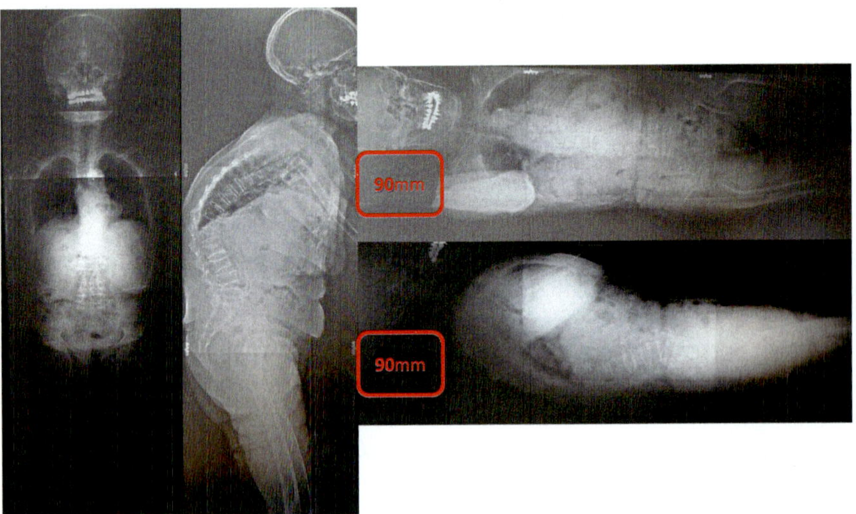

X-ray (X-P) images in the standing and recumbent postures
She needed a very high pillow due to her kyphosis

Fig. 1.13 Case 1. X-P images of the standing and recumbent postures in a patient with kyphosis

total score improved from 28 to 7, and NRS also decreased from 10 to 1 (Table 1.1). She said fine, “I am very happy that I can sleep better than a year ago. I feel refreshed. I can move my body enough. I find everything delicious.”

Case 2

A 48-year-old woman, height: 162.0 cm, and body weight: 51.0 kg. Neck pain appeared since the age of 28. She complains of bilateral upper extremity radiating pain and numbness, headache, and occipital pain upon waking since 45 years old.

She has neck pain since junior high school. She was treated for headache by a neurosurgeon, but it did not improve, so she visited our hospital. The type of pillow she had been using until then was a standard type and made of cotton. The height of the pillow was adjusted to 68 mm. Two weeks after the pillow adjustment, she was able to sleep well, and her neck pain and numbness in her upper limbs were reduced and the tension resolved. Three months later, the SSS-8 total score improved from 17 to 4 and the NRS decreased from 9 to 3 (Table 1.1). He said, “I satisfy the pillow therapy that has improved my cervical pain stiff shoulders and other symptoms.”

1.2.2.6 Discussion and Conclusion

By adjusting the height of the pillow to facilitate smooth turning, the patient was able to maintain good cervical spine and cervical spinal cord alignment, resulting in

Table 1.1 Case 1 and Case 2: The scores of SSS8, NRS and satisfaction

	SSS-8									
Case	Duration of pillow therapy	Stomach or bowel problems	Back pain	Pain in your arms, legs	Headache	Chest pain or shortness of breath	Dizziness	Feeling tired or having low	Trouble sleeping	Total score
Case 1	0	3	4	4	4	1	4	4	4	28
	2 W	2	3	4	1	0	1	2	4	17
	3 M	1	1	1	2	0	0	1	1	7
Case 2	0	2	4	4	2	0	0	1	4	17
	2 W	1	3	2	0	0	0	1	1	8
	3 M	0	1	1	0	1	0	0	1	4

Questionnaire			
NRS, pain intensity: 0 (no pain)–10 (worst possible pain)	Health condition: 0 (worst)–10 (best)	A 7-point rating scale for symptom improvement: 1 (very much improved)–7 (worse than ever)	A 4-point rating scale for treatment satisfaction: 1 (highly satisfied)–4 (highly dissatisfied)
10	10		
4	8	1	1
1	8	1	1
9	1		
4	4	2	1
3	4	2	1

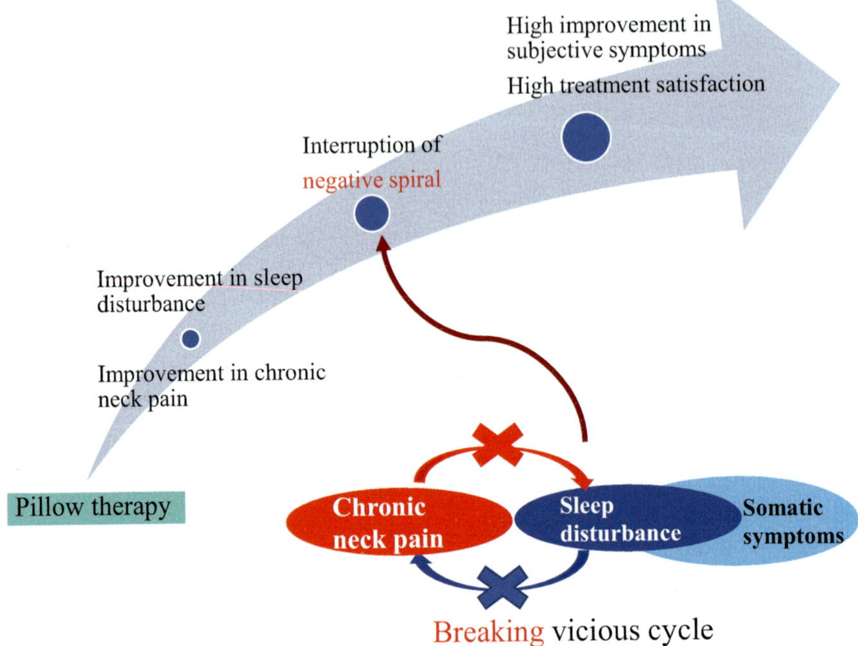

Fig. 1.14 Mechanism of action on pillow therapy

improvement of intractable neck pain and stiff shoulders with somatic symptoms within short or medium term. This trend was particularly pronounced in severe cases. These results suggest that breaking the vicious cycle between chronic neck pain and somatic symptoms including sleep disturbances can lead to a clear improvement in subjective symptoms and treatment satisfaction (Fig. 1.14).

Subsequently, we performed additional analyses of this study using different statistical methods. Changes over time in neck pain, assessed by NRS, and SSS-8 scores were analyzed using the Jonckheere-Terpstra test to determine whether pillow treatment relieved clinical symptoms. The clinical outcome of this study was the achievement of the minimal clinically important difference (MCID) in neck pain NRS and patient satisfaction at the end of 3-month treatment period. For the results and conclusions, see the authors' paper [10].

References

1. Safiri S, Kolahi A-A, Hoy D, Buchbinder R, Mansournia MA, Bettampadi D, et al. Global, regional, and national burden of neck pain in the general population, 1990-2017: systematic analysis of the global burden of disease study 2017. BMJ. 2020;368:m791. https://doi.org/10.1136/bmj.m791.
2. Kim SH, Lee DH, Yoon KB, An JR, Yoon DM. Factors associated with increased risk for clinical insomnia in patients with chronic neck pain. Pain Physician. 2015;18(6):593–8.

3. Chung K-F, Tso K-C. Relationship between insomnia and pain in major depressive disorder: a sleep diary and actigraphy study. Sleep Med. 2010;11(8):752–8.
4. Asih S, Neblett R, Mayer TG, Brede E, Gatchel RJ. Insomnia in a chronic musculoskeletal pain with disability population is independent of pain and depression. Spine J. 2014;14(9):2000–7.
5. O'Brien EM, Waxenberg LB, Atchison JW, Gremillion HA, Staud RM, McCrae CS, et al. Intraindividual variability in daily sleep and pain ratings among chronic pain patients: bidirectional association and the role of negative mood. Clin J Pain. 2011;27(5):425–33.
6. Kelly GA, Blake C, Power CK, O'Keeffe D, Fullen BM. The association between chronic low back pain and sleep a systematic review. Clin J Pain. 2011;27(2):169–81.
7. Artner J, Cakir B, Spiekermann J-A, Kurz S, Leucht F, Reichel H, et al. Prevalence of sleep deprivation in patients with chronic neck and back pain: a retrospective evaluation of 1016 patients. J Pain Res. 2013;6:1–6.
8. Bilterys T, Siffain C, De Maeyer I, Van Looveren E, Mairesse O, Nijs J, et al. Associates of Insomnia in people with chronic spinal pain: a systematic review and meta-analysis. J Clin Med. 2021;10(14):3175. https://doi.org/10.3390/jcm10143175.
9. Henningsen P, Zipfel S, Herzog W. Management of functional somatic syndromes. Lancet. 2007;369(9565):946–55.
10. Yamada S, Hoshi T, Toda M, Tsuge T, Matsudaira K, Oka H. Changes in neck pain and somatic symptoms before and after the adjustment of the pillow height. J Phys Ther Sci. 2023;35(2):106–13.

2 What Is the Reason Why Pillow Therapy Is Needed Now?

Abstract

This chapter first discusses what a pillow is, then defines pillow therapy and explains the purpose of sleep posture adjustment. We will explain how orthopedic surgeons and other clinicians should integrate pillow therapy into their daily practice. Conversely, it is important to know the limitations of pillow therapy to understand the correct use.

We will also present the timing for determining the effectiveness of pillow therapy, or other possible causes in cases not improved with pillow alone. Pillow therapy has three needs, i.e., social, patient, and physician needs. Even though there are differences in social and medical conditions and diseases in each country or region, these needs for pillow therapy always exist.

Next, we compare research on pillow around the world with those in Japan. The term "Cervical Pillow" has been spontaneously created without clear-cut definition and is being overused. We discuss how such research has influenced the currently marketed pillows.

We outline the history of our own pillow research and pillow-based empiric therapy and help you to imagine what our outpatient pillow clinic, named " The Pillow Clinic," doing the therapy.

Keywords

Pillow · Pillow therapy · Ruth Jackson MD · Cervical pillow · The pillow clinic · Empiric therapy

Supplementary Information The online version contains supplementary material available at https://doi.org/10.1007/978-981-99-0463-1_2.

S. Yamada, *Orthopaedic Pillow*, https://doi.org/10.1007/978-981-99-0463-1_2

2.1 What Is Pillow Therapy?

2.1.1 Definition of Pillow Therapy

Pillow therapy is a treatment to improve or resolve pain and/or somatic symptoms by using a pillow adjusted to the individual's physique.

2.1.2 What Is a Pillow?

We have no conscious control over our sleep posture during sleeping. Our sleeping posture is almost always determined by the bedding we selected. In brief, our choice of bedding determines our sleeping posture. There are many items that can regulate our sleep posture, such as pillows, sleeping bunks (beds and mattresses or Futons [Japanese-style mattress]), comforters, and pajamas. Out of them, the most significant influence element on sleep posture is pillow (Fig. 2.1). A slight change in pillow height affects not only the static posture (supine or lateral position) but also the ease of turning over in sleep (dynamic posture). Turning over is physiological response but an essential. I consider it important to be able to continue deep sleep without arousal when turning over. To achieve that, it is necessary to turn over smoothly with minimum energy. In conclusion, sleep posture adjustment is to maintain optimal static and dynamic posture during sleep, recover from physical and mental fatigue, and improve various symptoms, by using a pillow adjusted to each patient's age, gender, height, weight, shoulder width, and postural characteristics, such as kyphosis. Therefore, we believe that pillows should be regarded as "therapeutic tools" (Fig. 2.2).

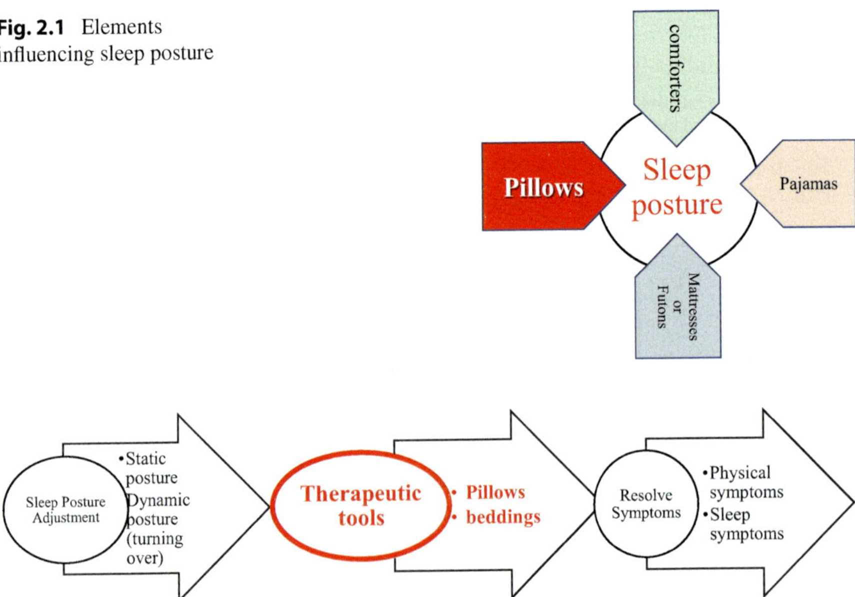

Fig. 2.1 Elements influencing sleep posture

Fig. 2.2 Pillows should be regarded as "therapeutic tools"

2.1.3 Positioning of Pillow Therapy

Positioning of the pillow therapy in daily practice depends on the physician's practice and/or therapeutic strategy. To explain our therapy I want to use orthopedics as an example, while it may vary from department to department. In orthopedics, following interview, palpation, and various laboratory testing, a diagnosis is made and treatment is started. A part of the treatments is educational lifestyle guidance for patient. One of the guidance is postural guidance. The management of posture should distinguish between daytime and nighttime. In the daytime, we can manage the posture by our own intention. However, in the nighttime, since we are unconscious, our sleep posture is almost determined by the bedding. It means your sleep posture is determined by the bedding you have chosen. In other words, bedding adjustment is the very posture management. Postural management is the basis or infrastructure, for any treatments, while there are a variety of treatment options. For example, even though a patient with cervical pain takes analgesics and undergoes rehabilitation in the daytime to make improve his/her symptoms, but the symptoms must flare up the next morning, as his/her sleeping posture is poor due to an ill-fitting pillow. Pillow adjustment is an essential part of the orthopedic infrastructure to improve symptoms, maintain good condition, and prevent flare-ups. Figure 2.3 indicates the positioning of pillow therapy in the orthopedic practice.

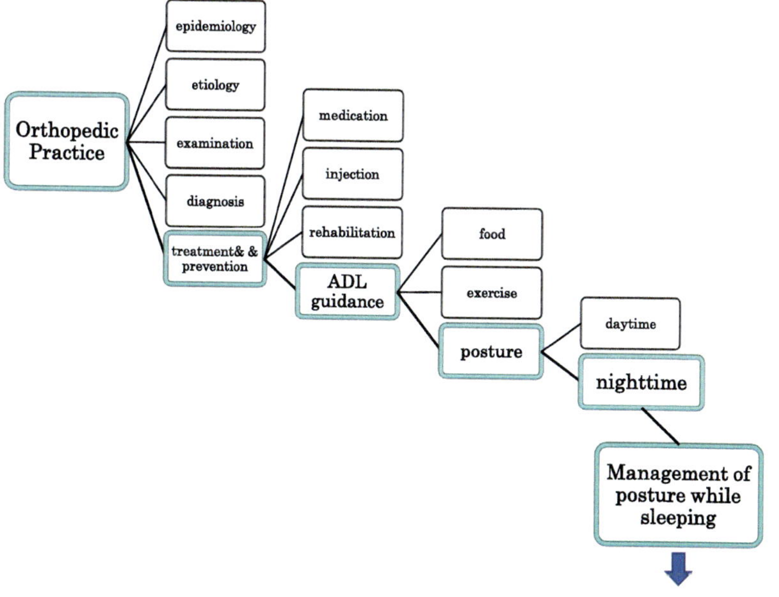

Fig. 2.3 Positioning of pillow therapy in orthopedic practice

2.1.4 Limitations of Pillow Therapy

Pillow therapy has of course limitations. It is not yet completely revealed how much it is effective for what symptoms, but let's try first the pillow therapy as an infrastructure (basic therapy) to the indications showing later. The onset of the effect of pillow therapy is rather quick, and in most cases, improvement can be seen a day after start using or within 2 weeks to 3 months at the latest. Conversely, in case the appropriate pillow is used, it is very rare to take several months for the effect being manifested. If the expected results are not confirmed, as the therapy is infrastructure, we should combine other treatments. Since the purpose of pillows is to improve postural adjustment, i.e., physical conditions, they may have limited efficacy to psychological or emotional symptoms. It is not difficult to determine the limits of effectiveness.

Despite using the suitably adjusted pillow, if a patient complains of "taking a long time to fall asleep (sleep onset disorder)," "waking up several times during the night (mid-night awakening)," "waking up more than two hours earlier than planned (early morning awakening)," or "not feeling like a good night's sleep (sound sleep disorder)," the patient's sleep disorders must be not caused by the pillow (sleep posture) but other reasons. Each of above mentioned four sleep disorders has its own causes. Depending on the cause, a consultation with a different specialist is necessary. For example, the common causes of mid-wake are adult diseases (e.g., hypertension, diabetes, etc.), sleep apnea syndrome, and depression. A patient should see a cardiologist for hypertension, a metabolic physician for diabetes, a respiratory physician or otolaryngologist for sleep apnea, and a psychiatrist or psychosomatic medicine for depression.

However, in our Pillow Clinical practice, we have experienced a number of patients who treated by their appropriate pillows also improved their complications such as hypertension and sleep apnea syndrome. Various symptoms that occur during sleep, such as pain, sleep disturbance, circulatory disturbance, respiratory condition, and psychosomatic disorder, may be not independent but affecting each other. The critical aspect is to start with safe, minimally invasive, and reasonable treatments as much as possible. Then, we carefully monitor the patient's progress, determine the limits of therapy, and if necessary, guide them to alternative treatments.

2.1.5 The Need for Pillow Therapy

As we mentioned before, pillow therapy has three kinds of needs (Fig. 2.4). These are social needs, patient needs, and physician needs. We described each of these needs and discuss the need for therapeutic pillows in modern medical care.

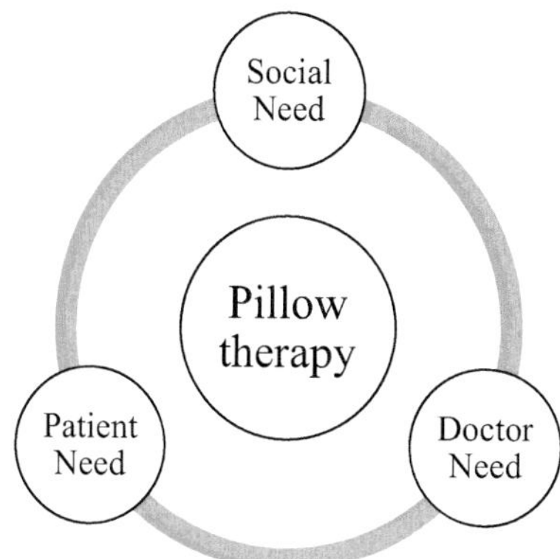

Fig. 2.4 Three need for pillow therapy

2.1.5.1 Social Needs

The Organisation for Economic Co-operation and Development (OECD) has ranked the Health Spendings (US dollars/capita) of countries in the world. In 2010–2020, the USA ranks first with 10.95 K, Switzerland second with 7.14 K, and Norway third with 6.75 K [1]. The health spending in each country has been increasing steadily year by year, and many countries have renewed their highest record in 2020. Especially under the current global outbreak of COVID-19, countries are forced to reconsider where to prioritize the investment of any healthcare resources, including healthcare spending, medical manpower, medical technologies, and so on. Japanese Health Spending is ranked 14th in the world at 4.69 K US dollars/capita [1].

It is generally said that the reasons for the increase in health spending are the aging of population and the advancement of medical technologies but peculiarly Japanese factors include high drug prices, high drug user fees, and high medical material prices. In order to maintain the National Health Insurance System, which could go bankrupt if left inaction, we should create "an infrastructure for health not relying on medicines or medical products." Health insurance systems vary from country to country, and there are disparities in the services that people can receive. Many people would prefer lower-cost, effective healthcare solutions. Examples of such treatments include presymptomatic or preventive medicine restoring daily physical and mental health through good sleep, and pain control without using medicines. Sleep posture management by pillow therapy is safe, effective, simple, and low cost, in other words, it is in line with the need of the current society.

2.1.5.2 Patient Needs

Needless to say, patients visit medical institutions to want to be relieved from the difficult symptoms. Patients' requests like medications, injections, rehabilitation, etc., are all a method, not the ultimate goal for the treatment. The goal is "to be free from symptoms." However, in actual clinical environments, it seems that many

No	age	1.Male 2.femake	length of attendance (Month)	Number of clinics attended ※
1	43	1	2	1
2	55	1	96	2
3	66	1	36	1
4	46	2	2	1
5	50	1	15	2
6	64	1	4	2
7	49	2	288	1
8	49	1	360	2
9	64	1	216	2
10	69	1	12	2
11	45	2	372	1
13	67	1	61	2
14	62	2	432	1
15	31	2	5	1
16	83	2	3	4
17	74	2	240	1
18	62	1	26	
19	61	2	72	1
20	48	1	32	2
21	46	2	123	1
22	50	2	36	1
23	51	2	24	4
24	35	2	120	2
25	50	2	35	3
26	41	1	6	1
27	51	2	312	2
28	50	1	24	2
29	50	2	15	1
30	75	2	4	2

60 of the 84 patients who came to my clinic with chronic neck pain had attended other clinics (table shows selected 30 example cases)

Orthopedics	47
Neurosurgery	12
Pain clinic	3
Psychiatry/psychosomatic medicine	8
Sleep medicine	6
Acupuncture, moxibustion, osteopathy, chiropractic	8
Total	60

The average length of attendance was 8.8 years

※Indicates the number of clinics the patient has visited in the past, excluding our clinic

Fig. 2.5 History of visits to other hospitals and clinics

treatments do not set the ultimate goal to "curing." To be more specific, "There is no abnormality in the X-ray, so there is no problem," "It can't be helped because you are old," or "prescribing a poultice to ease one's mind" must not solve any problem. It should be the other way around. We have to positively resolve the complaint that is troubling the patient because X-ray did not indicate any abnormalities, the patient is elderly, or no definitive diagnosis was able to be made. It is no overstatement that the persistence of such physical and/or mental complaints (including some indefinite complaints) impairs the patient's health and that leads to significant social and economic losses.

In fact, in patient survey of our Pillow Clinic conducted in 2014, there were 84 patients with chronic neck pain as their main complaint who eventually reached our clinic. 60 of the 84 patients had been visiting a number of medical centers one after another for an average duration of 8.8 years and having received various treatments (Fig. 2.5). After only 2 weeks of the pillow therapy, many of those patients experienced significant improvement in their symptoms. Not a few of them commented, "I can go to school again," "I can go to work again," or "I can go back into the community." It is the duty of the therapist to understand the true needs of the patient and provide an appropriate solution. Pillow therapy is one of the beneficial solutions to reach the final goal, even if the patient does not know or has never experienced it (subclinical needs).

2.1.5.3 Doctor Needs

As of January 2022, there are more than 60 medical institutions in Japan that agree with our pillow therapy and have introduced the Pillow Clinic system in their own institutes. In addition, the number of orthopedic surgeons and clinicians who use the Orthopedic Pillow has increased to more than 500 (including professors and associate professors at university medical schools). Those numbers have been increasing every year. Many doctors ask us, "I have asked by patients what kind of pillow they should use," "I want to know what kind of pillow I should recommend to my patients," "Can I recommend a commercially available contour pillow to my patients?" As there are many kinds of pillows on the market and abundant information about pillows, patients are confused about the choice and ask their doctors. However, doctors have poor knowledge of medically proper pillows, so they are at a loss to answer the question. Many doctors and medical professionals want to know "the standard of the correct pillow" and it is the doctor's needs.

2.2 Comparison of Pillow Research in the World and Pillow Therapy in Japan

In this chapter, we discuss the gaps in pillow research between Japan and overseas, and how they have effected marketed pillows.

2.2.1 Dr. Ruth Jackson MD, Pioneer of Pillow Research

As far as we know, the first person to seriously study pillows and actually develop her own pillow was Dr. Ruth Jackson MD (1902–1994, USA). She was the first female member of the American Academy of Orthopaedic Surgeons (AAOS) and the specialist of cervical spine developing the Jackson's compression test, the famous test for the diagnosis of cervical spondylotic radiculopathy. She later founded the Ruth Jackson Orthopaedic Society. It is impossible to understand the medical history of the pillow without knowing her researches on the cervical spine and her major papers and books. Unfortunately, I am currently unable to obtain a paper of the original work in 1949, "The Cervical Syndrome." I have found the following articles, the second Edition in1958 [2] and fourth Edition in1977 [3] of the Cervical Syndrome published by CHARLES C THOMAS Springfield, Illinois, USA.

She first used the term "Cervical Pillow" in 1949 and recommended the use of the cervical roll pillow that she developed. The reason why she called it "the cervical roll pillow" or "cervical contour pillow" can be inferred from the following statement: "By a process of trial and error, the Cervical Contour Pillow was developed. It should be stuffed with feathers and down or with Dacron. When in use it should be flattened in the center so that the neck rests on the proper amount of support for comfort. This leaves bulge on either side which prevents too much rotation and lateral bending. If patients sleep on his side the bulge at either end gives adequate support to assure comfort and to keep the neck straight" [2, 3]. Comparing the photographs and X-ray images in the supine position without the pillow, with the Ordinary Pillow, and with The Cervical Contour Pillow, it was only a normal forward curve of the neck and no hyperextension when the Cervical Contour Pillow was used. This is the most comfortable sleeping or supine position. She concluded "The Cervical Contour Pillow has been one of the greatest adjuncts in the treatment of cervical nerve root irritation, and in many cases no other treatment is needed" [2, 3].

Jackson's pillow has been commercially available, and as long ago as 1967, Cervipillo® (TRU-EZE Mfg. Co., Inc.) was listed in the brochure of the International Congress of ORTHOTICS AND PROSTHETICS held in Miami, along with X-ray images of using pillow [4].

In the process of researching these old articles I came across an incomprehensible article. This Classic article is a reprint of the original work by Ruth Jackson, MD, FACS, The Cervical Syndrome in 1949 [5].

The article stated "The author designed a special pillow which has been the greatest adjunct in treatment. The pillow fits the normal contour of the neck and keeps the neck straight while the patient is sleeping (see Figs. 5A-B, 6B′P.1744 in [5]). The conventional pillow causes flexion of the neck (see Fig. 6A-A′P.1744 in [5]) and aggravates the symptoms." The statement "In the X-ray image, the neck became straight using the Contour pillow in the supine position and neck flection using the conventional pillow" is inconsistent with the view in her original paper "a normal forward curve using the Contour pillow and flection using a conventional pillow." I don't know if this is a work error by the editor in reprint. I would speculate that the Cervical Contour Pillow causes cervical forward curve, which is the idealistic view of Ruth Jackson MD. In the original "The Cervical Syndrome," the cervical spine was cervical forward curve in the model used in the photographs, but it was not clearly stated whether it was cervical forward curve in other models of different physiques. In other words, the Cervical Contour Pillow of a given height and size could be higher or lower for each model, depending on the physique of the different models in the photographs. This would have also changed the alignment of the neck, so that in one X-ray the model's cervical spine would have been kyphotic and in another model's X-ray the cervical spine would have been straight. I sent an email query to the editor of this issue of Clinical Orthopaedics and Related Research in 2021, but did not receive an appropriate response, so this issue is no longer a matter of conjecture.

Her paper and words were subsequently cited in many articles on pillows [6–12]. For example, "One of the most important factors in appropriate pillow selection is adequate support of cervical lordosis, and a major role of pillows is to support and maintain the cervical spine in a neutral position during sleep" [11]. "According to a previous case study using lateral radiographs of the cervical spine with and without exposure to regular and roll-shaped pillows, the roll-shaped pillow restored cervical lordosis and decreased neck pain and discomfort while sleeping (Jackson 2010)" [10]. Most were interpreted as Jackson stated that the cervical spine becomes lordotic when using a cervical roll pillow [10, 12]. Susan J Gordon said "The contour foam pillow supports the cervico-thoracic spine any differently to a regular-shaped foam pillow when side lying" [13–15]. Conversely, some articles denying the efficacy of Ruth Jackson's cervical contour pillow have also been published: "During the course of the roll pillow trial, 10 subjects dropped out during the trial period and gave uniformly negative comments regarding the roll pillow" [16].

Interestingly, he also published a number of Jackson Cervipillow and many contour pillow designations and their respective suppliers around 1997 [16]. I have not been able to find most of them on the internet as of 2021.

2.2.2 Recent Worldwide Pillow Researches: Three Discussion Points

2.2.2.1 Point 1: Shortage of Research on Pillows for Management of Nocturnal Cervical Spine Posture in Orthopedic Surgery

Many articles have pointed out that exacerbation or relief of neck pain and arm pain depends on pillows used at night [5–9, 11–19] and therefore pillows are recognized as one of the prevention and treatment tools of neck pain [20, 21]. Since 1990, number of reports on pillow has been increasing in the areas of ergonomics, medical engineering, public health, physiotherapy, and chiropractic. Particularly, Susan J Gordon, a physiotherapy clinician, has published many high-quality papers on research methods for pillows [13–15, 17, 22]. Conversely, clinical research reports on pillows published by orthopedic surgeons and prosthetist are rare [5, 19]. Although many orthopedic surgeons have realized that neck pain onsets from malposture and mainly pay attention to postural management, such as standing and sitting during the daytime, they have paid little attention to cervical spine postural management during sleep, because patients are unconscious during sleep and cannot adjust their cervical posture consciously. As many papers have pointed out that the shape, height, and material of the pillow affect the alignment of the cervical and thoracic spine [6, 13, 23], it is thought that bedding adjustment plays an important role in the management of cervical spine posture during sleep.

2.2.2.2 Point 2: The Definition of Cervical Pillow Is Unclear

As mentioned before, the terminology of “Cervical Pillow,” advocated by Ruth Jackson in 1949, has been seen in clinical studies using pillows since 1990 [6, 8, 9, 11, 18, 19, 24]. However, its concept, size, shape, and material vary widely and no common concept or definition has established yet. In other words, clinicians or researchers merely use the term “cervical pillow” in a sense of their own understood. In a systematic review by Nora Shields et al. [25] in 2006 on cervical pillows for neck pain, they concluded that there were insufficient evidence to determine whether the Cervical Pillow can reduce chronic neck pain or not. They also stated that a high-quality randomized controlled trial should be required prior to recommending the use of “cervical pillows,” which is still undefined and not yet fully validated, in clinical practice.

Following this publication of the systematic review, a number of reports have been published on the pillow by many researchers. In 2021, Johnson C.Y. Pang et al. [26] published a systematic review and meta-analysis on pillows in the Clinical Biomechanics. They collected 1236 of literatures on pillow published by September 2020 via the Physiotherapy Evidence Database (PEDro) and assessed their methodologies. The concept of key words for document retrieval was “pillow and pillow design" and "the effect of pillows on neck conditions and cervical spine symptoms." The collected studies were evaluated by their outcomes on pain, disability, pillow satisfaction, and sleep quality. Ultimately, only nine studies were evaluable with high quality. The result of the meta-analysis recommended the usage of rubber pillows with statistical significance. Comparing among different pillow materials, the rubber and spring pillows showed efficacies on chronic neck pain, arousal symptoms, neck disability, and satisfaction, except sleep quality. Conversely, no evidence supported the superiority of contour pillows to regular-shaped pillows on pain, neck problems, or sleep quality. Even based on the study results evaluated by this systematic review and meta-analysis, the Cervical Pillow was not able to define.

I agree definitely with their following statement in Discussion; "To prevent unnecessary stress on the cervical spine and restore proper spinal alignment during sleep, a suitable pillow is necessary to fit the individual's body structure" and "The cervical alignment (CA) may significantly change with the shape and height of the pillow rather than its material. However, knowledge of the optimal CA in the supine position remains limited." However, they seemed to presume the following information in Japan to be Takano's one; "Despite Takano (2018) recommending that the CA should be around 15° [27], there is no supporting scientific evidence." In fact, the Takano information they quoted was what I explained in a Japanese TV program and a figure created by a TV station (NHK, the Japan Broadcasting Corporation). In other words, the source of "CA is about 15°" is my research results explained in this book. As I had not published any English articles at that time, they might consider the evidence was "unspecified".

In their conclusion, they pointed out two issues: the effects of different shapes and heights of pillows on cervical alignment, and the optimal CA in the supine position was not yet clear. We had already revealed in the 1970s that the supine cervical tilt angle was approximately 15° irrespective of age and sex, based on accumulated clinical practice data of symptom improvement in patients. Further research is required to confirm whether the same results can be obtained in various racial groups with different body shapes and sizes, based on the "optimal pillow height for Japanese people is about 15°" that we have established. Only then will the definition of the Cervical Pillow be complete.

2.2.2.3 Point 3: Discussion of Pillow Shape, Material, and Height

Many studies reported on shapes of pillow, and contour pillows or shape pillows were common in ergonomic approach. Recently, there are dominantly two types of pillow shapes: the horizontal contour pillow that is high on both sides and low in the center, and the vertical contour pillow that is high under the neck and low at the top of the head when sleeping in the supine position.

First, the reason for recommending a horizontal contour pillow is that it is believed that the pillow should be higher to match the shoulder height in the side lying position, and that the pillow height should be different in the supine and side lying position [8, 28].

P. Erfanian [8] reported that as neck thickness and shoulder width are not equal, the heights of the pillow should change between back and side lying positions. He said that semi-custom pillows address this problem by using the lower center curve for back sleeping and the higher curve on either side for side sleeping. However in my opinion, we can determine one single height that is compatible with both supine and side lying positions in almost all cases, except for persons with special body shapes. Moreover, only finding this unique height can complete the smoothest turning. Typical examples of special body shapes are persons with particularly broad shoulders or severe kyphosis.

Dengchuan Cai et al. [28] reported that currently available pillows were too high for the supine position and too low for the side lying position. Furthermore, they stated that the pillow height differs considerably between the supine and side lying positions, so it is necessary to design a pillow that takes this into account. They found that the pillow heights for male were 3.7 cm and 14.8 cm for supine position and side lying position, respectively. In a similar way, for female were 2.5 cm and 11.5 cm, respectively. Therefore, when sleeping in the supine position, a neck rest should be considered for neck support. However, in comparison with the results of our studies, the pillow height in the side lying position is too high and it in the supine position was too low for both men and women. We consider neck rest is unnecessary once the unique one pillow height that is compatible with both supine and side lying positions is determined.

Second, the reason for recommending a vertical contour pillow is to support the curve of the neck [5, 10, 12, 24, 29]. However, the evidence is not sufficient from a clinical point of view. Shuo-Fang Liu et al. [29] reported that the most comfortable pillow was the "standard pillow," "cervical pillow," and "shoulder pillow." However, they excluded subjects who preferred to lie on their side during sleep, so this conclusion only applies to subjects who lie in the lateral position.

According to the results of Mi Yang Jeon et al. study [10], the orthopedic pillow consisted of 7 segments, each of them containing multiple capsules, and confirmed a significant increase in repeatedly measured cervical kyphosis compared to baseline cervical kyphosis measured in the standing with the neck in neutral position. Conversely, our studies have revealed that cervical spine alignment decreased lordosis and came closer straight when subjects with cervical pain used pillows adapted to their physique. In their experiment, the pillows were adapted only in the supine position, whereas in our experiment, the pillows were adapted in three conditions, including in the supine position, lateral position, and turning over. When optimizing all of the three conditions, the cervical spine alignment is expected to be near straight.

Since almost all researchers conduct their research using commercially available pillows that have different shapes, materials, and heights, it is impossible to compare and evaluate what parameter influenced the study outcome, the effects of pillows. I believe that the order of priority is important in setting the conditions of the pillow and the highest priority is pillow height, and then materials and shapes should be chosen to maintain that height. Some studies evaluated pillow heights that were the most important parameter [6, 8, 18, 24, 28, 30–32], but they compared in the unit of centimeter [6, 8, 31, 32] not in millimeter what we adjust precisely.

Sicong Ren et al. [6] used the four different heights pillows of 110 mm, 130 mm, 150 mm, 170 mm. P Erfanian et al. [8] let the subject choose a prototype (semi-customized) pillow, one of four pillows with different heights of 1 cm each instead of using a totally customized pillow. Hyung Cheol Kim [32] used three different pillow heights of flat (0 cm), 10 cm, and 20 cm pillows. Isabel C.N. Sacco et al. [31] used foam pillows of three different heights 5 cm, 10 cm, and 14 cm.

When it comes to the correlation between pillow heights and body physique, Jia-Chi Wang et al. [24] concluded the height of the best self-selected pillow did not correlate with anatomical parameters, including body weight, body length, BMI, neck length, and neck thickness. The optimal pillow height recommendations based on anatomical body measurements may be inappropriate. However, in our research, we found a strong correlation between body size parameters (body weight and height) and pillow height, because we used objective measurements (anatomical body measurements) of pillows rather than following subjects' preference. Conversely, Dengchuan Cai et al. [28] measured the 18 of body dimensions in the standard posture to determine the size of pillows. According to the results of their study, the key points for pillow design were derived: (1) Pillow height for the supine position and lateral position should be different. (2) Pillow height for the supine position and lateral position is 3.7 cm and 14.8 cm for male and 2.5 cm and 11.5 cm for female. Compared to our study, their pillow height for the lateral position is too high. One of the reasons may be that they measured "shoulder breadth maximum" and "width from neck to shoulder" in the standard posture (sitting or standing), which caused a difference from the actual sleeping posture. In fact, in the sleeping posture, the shoulder joint is not changed. In fact, in the sleeping posture, the shoulder joint moves forward from the torso, so that the shoulder width is narrower than in the sitting or standing position. The width of shoulder should be measured after turning over several times.

Jin-Gang Her et al. [30] tried to determine pillow designs suitable for supine and lateral positions. Thereby they created an air bag in the region that would contact the neck and measure the pressure to maintain the normal cervical lordotic curvature is 30° to 35°. I don't understand the need for direct pressure on neck, I believe that adjusting the pillow to the proper height will stabilize the neck without direct pressure on this part.

Juhyun Son et al. [33] systematically reviewed preceding studies on pillows, collected the data of more than 200 commercially available pillows, and classified pillows into six types according to its shape and contour. They also investigated the sleep habit and sleeping symptom of Korean adults relating to the comfort and support characteristics of pillows and the relationship between sleep quality and pillow design factors. As a conclusion, in order to reduce the negative symptoms of the head, neck, and shoulders, it was important to properly design pillow's shape. In cases of neck fatigue, it was desirable to design a pillow using materials such as latex or memory foam that have good neck support. In addition, to reduce neck fatigue and shoulder pain, it was necessary to consider the proper height of the neck support area in the lateral position.

I have doubt about conditions of the pillow used in this study. Subjects selected the pillow from six different types that were different in firmness and height. It means that the outcomes of subjects' comfort and degrees of support by pillow may be affected by not only shape but also height and firmness of pillows. In my opinion, each type of pillows should be evaluated at different heights and in both supine and lateral recumbent positions.

Why haven't researchers around the world noticed the important thing that a slight change in pillow height can result in an optimal cervical spine tilt angle in the supine position? Two reasons are speculated. First, many researchers, same as Dr. Ruth Jackson MD, may have believed that the ideal cervical spine alignment in the supine position is curvature, or curve, in the standing position, and not have come up with the idea that the straight cervical spine alignment can improve symptoms. Therefore, the idea of a constant angle between the straight cervical spine and the lying surface did not occur to them.

Second, as the priority was placed on the "shape" of the pillow to support the cervical spine, they may not have paid attention to the fact that the optimum angle for the cervical spine can be obtained by slight adjustment of the "height."

Figure 2.6 shows the cervical spine alignments in the supine position: no pillows or by different types of pillows. (a) No pillow: the cervical spine alignment is straight and the supine cervical tilt angle is almost zero degrees (Fig. 2.6a). (b) Ordinary pillow made by down or cotton: the cervical spine alignment depends on the degree of pillow compressed, and not constant of the cervical spine alignment (Fig. 2.6b). (c) Cervical contour pillow: the cervical alignment becomes lordosis when the contour pillow is fitted to the position of the head and neck. However, when the head position does not match the pillow, the alignment changes in various ways (Fig. 2.6c). (d) Our Orthopedic Pillow: the cervical spine alignment is near straight and it is about 15° at the optimal height of pillow (Fig. 2.6d). Figure 2.7 shows the cervical spine alignment in the lateral position: no pillows or by different types of pillows. (a) No pillow: the cervical spine alignment becomes severe flexion (Fig. 2.7a). (b) Ordinary pillow made by down or cotton: the cervical alignment is moderate flexion. However, the height of the pillow depends on the degree of pillow compressed (Fig. 2.7b). (c) Contour Pillow: the cervical spine alignment is in a slight flexion. However, when the contour pillow is not fitted to the position of the head and neck, the alignment changes in various ways (Fig. 2.7c). (d) Our Orthopedic Pillow: the cervical spine alignment is straight, and the lying surface and the head and neck axis become parallel. Even in other persons, if the pillow height is optimal for each individual, the axis of the head and neck is aligned in parallel with the bed surface (Fig. 2.7d).

We have set the priority of requirements in choosing a pillow. First, determine the optimum height, then select the material to maintain the height, and finally the shape for easy turning over. If the pillow doesn't fit, the height is adjusted first, followed by adjustment of the hardness. It is important to note that if you make the pillow too soft, the pillow sinks beyond the allowance range, 5 mm, and not to be the optimal height.

If you change the height, hardness, and material of the pillow at the same time, it is hard to identify what caused unfit.

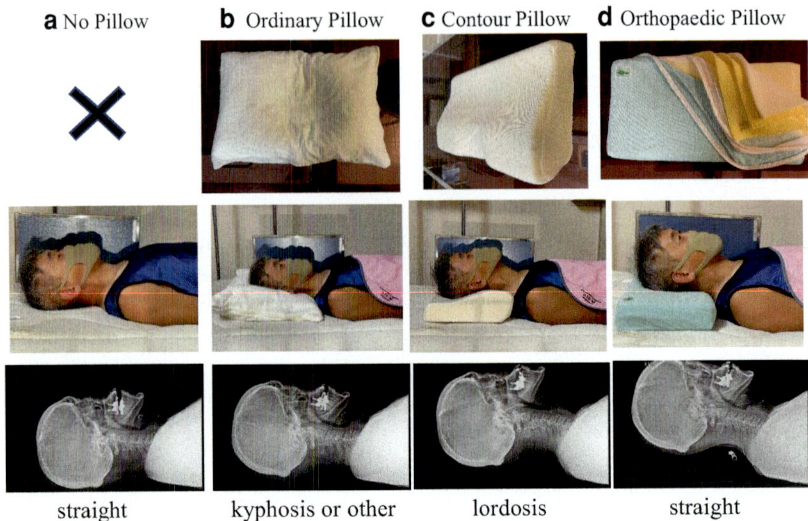

Fig. 2.6 Cervical spine alignments by pillow types in the supine position. (**a**) No pillow. (**b**) Ordinary pillow. (**c**) Contour pillow. (**d**) Orthopedic pillow

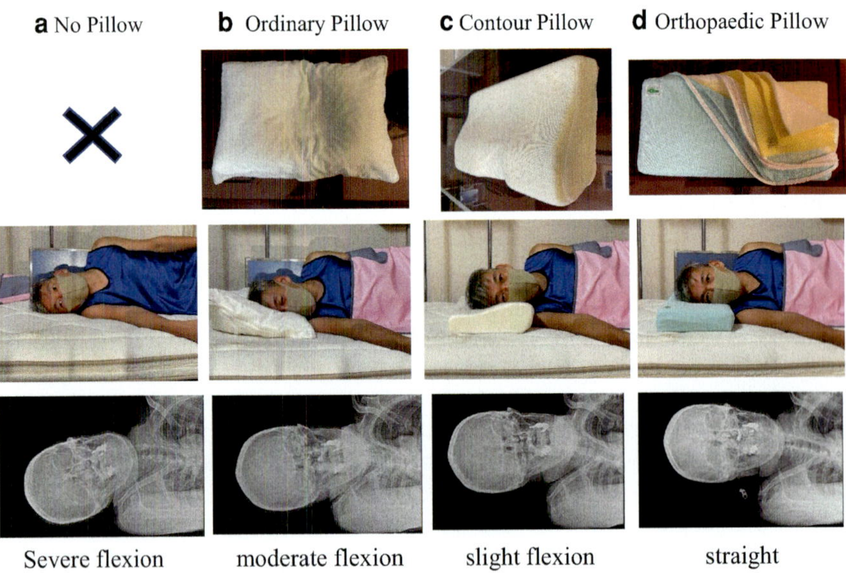

Fig. 2.7 Cervical spine alignments by pillow types in the lateral position. (**a**) No pillow. (**b**) Ordinary pillow. (**c**) Contour pillow. (**d**) Orthopedic pillow

2.2.3 The History of Our Research and Empirical Medicine on Pillow

In 1971, Dr. Hidemaru Kumagai, my father and the previous director of our clinic, established Naruse Orthopaedic Clinic in Tokyo, Japan. There, he began clinical research on pillows, but it was not of a quality that could be called research at the time. He had patients with cervical spondylosis bring Zabuton (Japanese floor cushion stuffed with cotton or wool) and cotton blanket with them as materials for making pillows. He made a tailored pillow cutting and layering these materials to fit each patient's physique and adjusted the height of the pillow. He monitored the adaptation of the pillow and the progress of the symptoms for long period. Through his repeated pillow adjustments for many patients, he had established a unique pillow adjustment method. In 2002, about 30 years later, I modified the method and perfected the Set-up for Spinal Sleep (SSS) Method, and I have been using the SSS method in my Pillow clinic in 16 Gou Orthopaedic Clinic since 2007 for treatment. Using this method, a pillow that fits individual's physique can be easily made from materials that are found anywhere in the house, i.e., Japanese doormats (placing inside the door of a house made by cotton, wool, or linen) and cotton blankets (Fig. 2.8). Details are shown in Sect. 4.4.

After graduating from Showa University School of Medicine, my father trained in the Department of Orthopaedic Surgery at Showa University Hospital before opening his own clinic. At the university hospital, he was a member of the research team for the cervical spine and conducted animal experiments on the cervical intervertebral disc. The history of our pillow research began with empiric medicine to determine how to adjust pillows to improve patients' symptoms and then conducted basic and clinical research to elucidate and verify the mechanism. Since there was no preceding research in Japan at that time, we constructed a theory based on the facts only, i.e., observations in clinical practice. In recent years, researchers can refer to preceding studies and use the shapes and materials of commercially available pillows used by their predecessors. Therefore, current researchers seem to be overly preoccupied with preconceived ideas and, in a sense, they seem to be writing papers based on ideal experimental results that are convenient. Essentially, the pursuit of truth in clinical practice means observing changes in patients' symptoms, accumulating scientific verifications, and elucidating new truths. Sometimes, the truth is a novel outcome that no one predicted and may rewrite the conventional facts.

The reports on pillow that my father and I have conducted in our clinic are listed in comparison with some papers from overseas in Table 2.1. Researches on pillow have been conducted in Australia, Korea, Taiwan, Canada, China, USA, Brazil, Iran, and so on. The research fields included physiology, engineering, ergonomics, physiotherapy, chiropractic, and medical engineering, with most studies conducted by specialists such as physiotherapists, chiropractors, nurses, and engineers, and very few studies conducted by orthopedic (spine and joint surgery) surgeons. The research interests of international researchers are

Since 1971
Naruse Orthopaedic Clinic
at Tokyo, Japan

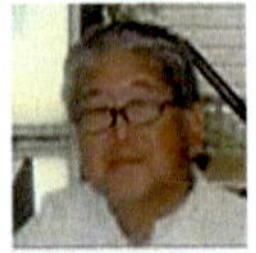

Since 2007
16 Gou Orthopaedic Clinic
at Kanagawa, Japan

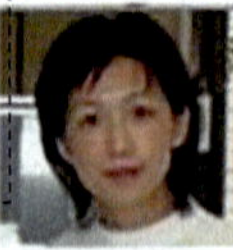

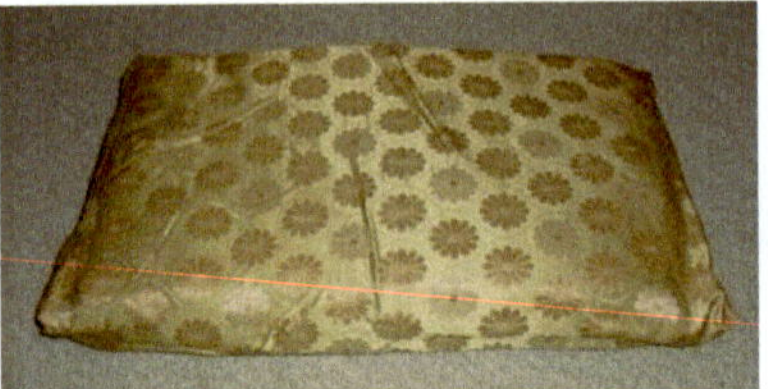

Version1: a pillow made of Zabuton (Japanese floor cushion)

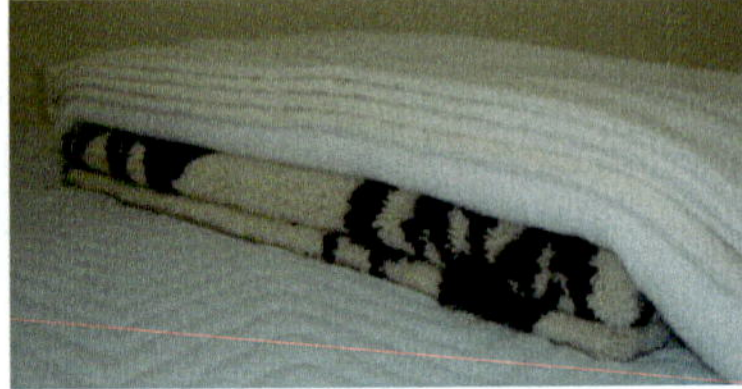

Version2: a pillow made of Japanese entrance mat (lower) and Towelket (upper)

Fig. 2.8 Two handmade pillows. We have made the handmade pillows for over 60,000 patients

Table 2.1 Comparison of foreign literature and authors' ideas in pillow research

	Papers in English (mainly since 1990)	Our reports
Country	Australia, Korea, Taiwan, Canada, China, USA, Brazil, Iran, etc.	Japan
Field of research	Physiology, ergonomics, physiotherapy, chiropractic, biological sciences, medical engineering	Orthopedics
Researcher(s)	Physiotherapists, chiropractors, nurses, engineers	Orthopedic surgeon
Interests	Pillow design, comfort, head and neck pressure, cervical alignment, neck pain, sleep quality	Clinical symptoms (neck pain, etc.), spinal alignment
Subjects	Asymptomatic adults, mostly aged 20–40 years	Complainants, from 10s to 80s
Assessment method	VAS, NDI, sleep questionnaire, satisfaction scale	VAS, NRS, SSS8, X-P, MRI
Key parameters for pillows	Material, shape, and temperature	Optimum height (smoothest turning), firmness, and shape
Pillow materials	Latex, low rebound, high resilience, polyurethane foam, feathers, plastic chips, etc.	Urethane foam, chip urethane, polyethylene, etc.
Pillow height in comparison	Every 5 cm (e.g., 5, 10, 14 cm)	Every 5 mm (e.g., 60, 65, 70 mm)
Pillow shape	1. Contour pillow with high sides and low center • Pillow height differs between supine and side lying positions 2. Contour pillow low at the top and high under the neck • Supports the curve of the neck	Flat (at optimal height) • Shoulders move flexibly when turning over • No need to curve the neck • At optimal height the neck is straight
Prospects	Necessity of RCT	Necessity of RCT

mostly in pillow design, comfort, and sleep quality, followed by head and neck pressure, cervical alignment, and cervical pain. However, we have studied patient symptoms such as pain, stiffness, numbness, and various disorders. In other countries, most of the study subjects are healthy volunteers, asymptomatic adults, and people aged 20s to 40s, and there are few studies on patients with complaints or symptoms like ours.

Since we regard pillows as a therapeutic tool, our research subjects are usually patients, who have visited the Pillow Clinic or those who are with symptoms and/or complaints. Our database includes from children under 10 years old to elders over 80 years old. The VAS (Visual Analogue Scale), NDI (Neck Disability Index), Sleep Questionnaire, Satisfaction Scale, etc. are used mainly for evaluation out of Japan. We also use subjective evaluation items such as NRS (Numerical Rating Scale) and SSS-8 (Somatic Symptom Scale8), but we also use objective evaluation such as X-ray images and MRI imaging. Next, on pillows. in other countries, the key parameters on a pillow are material, shape, temperature, etc., but the first priority is materials. Initially, they consider what kind of material to use. The characteristics of material, its feeling, and comfort are taking account. Then, they consider what shape is suitable for that material. Conversely, as we are most concerned with the pillow height fitting to the individual's physique, we choose a material that provides the proper height, and shape that is firm enough that the height will remain the same even after all night use. The priority of the parameters focusing on is quite difference between overseas researchers and us. In other countries, the shape of the pillow is determined by observing only the supine and lateral positions in the static sleep posture. However, we believe that a pillow should be adaptable supine and lateral positions not only in the static sleep posture, but also in the dynamic sleep posture, i.e., turning over.

We have been continuously advocating the importance of turning over when considering sleep posture, since we started the Pillow Clinic in 2002. In recent years, many marketed pillows and bedding products have claimed that turning over is important. Unfortunately, however, many of these products do not actually allow for smooth turning over. We purchased commercially available pillows of typical shapes and actually checked their ability to turning over in sleep (Fig. 2.9, Videos 2.1, 2.2, 2.3, and 2.4). In other words, there is a discrepancy between product advertisements and actual effects.

In comparison to the research on pillows of ours with those of overseas, basic stances are very difference. We have pillows that specifically developed to improve or resolve patients' symptoms since more than 50 years. A lot of clinical experience has already been accumulated in which patients with cervical spine symptoms have been improved by using the pillow. Based on these experiences, we have conducted several basic and clinical studies to elucidate the mechanism of this pillow. In contrast, most of the studies in overseas used the pillow evaluated in the preceding studies or marketed pillows as research materials and formulated an ideal hypothesis first then verify it. Therefore, so many parameters (material, height, hardness, shape, design, etc.) should be evaluated in the study, and the priority in selecting or

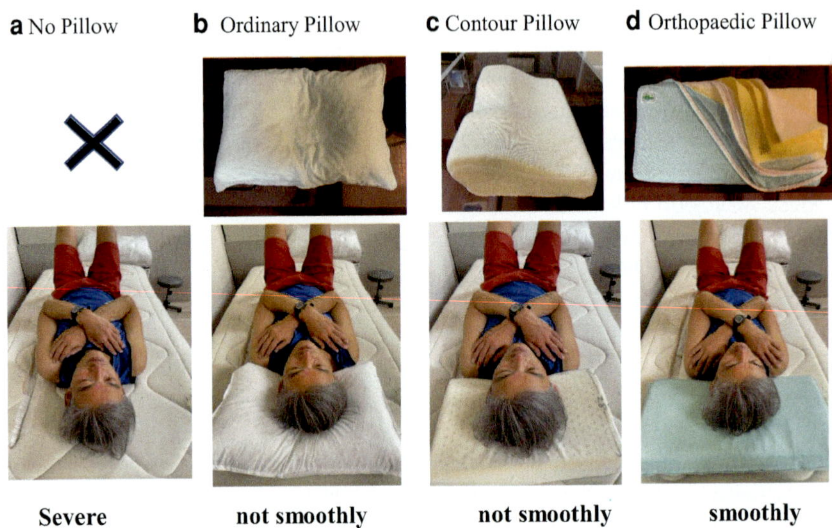

Fig. 2.9 Differences of turning over by pillow types (movie). (**a**) No pillow. (**b**) Ordinary pillow. (**c**) Contour pillow. (**d**) Orthopedic pillow

designing a pillow was not clear. As a result, it is often unclear which parameters contributed significantly to the outcomes. However, for both parties, in the future, randomized controlled trials (RCTs) are needed to validate the efficacy of pillows for treatment.

2.3 The Pillow Clinic

2.3.1 What Is the Pillow Clinic?

In recent years, many "specialized outpatient clinics" have been opened in Japan. Names of typical outpatient clinic/department include internal medicine, surgery, orthopedics, otolaryngology, ophthalmology, pediatrics, obstetrics and gynecology, and psychiatry, but a specialized outpatient clinic is an outpatient clinic conducted by an expert in concerned field with the aim of promoting the targeted disease or treatment. For example, they specify the name of the disease like "outpatient clinic specializing in headache," "outpatient clinic specializing in dizziness," "outpatient clinic specializing in asthma," and "outpatient clinic specializing in dementia," or the name of target patients like "outpatient clinic specializing in gender difference," "outpatient clinic specializing in puberty," and "outpatient clinic specializing in menopause." Patients can select a specialized outpatient clinic according to their signs or symptoms.

In 2002, we established an outpatient clinic specializing in treatment with pillows, named "The Pillow Clinic." Once again, the definition of the Pillow Clinic is "an outpatient clinic that aims to improve various physical and/or mental symptoms by adjusting pillows." Pillow adjustment is performed using materials that patients bring into. Specifically, the physician examines the patient and diagnoses symptoms or diseases. If the symptom or disease is caused by improper sleep posture, or if it is caused by something else but the improper sleep posture is thought to be an aggravating factor, a pillow adjustment is indicated. However, the range of indication for pillow adjustment can be considered more broadly. Even though a patient has a physical or mental disorder, "good sleep" is a basic and fundamental factor for recovery. It is the very infrastructure of treatment. From this point of view, we believe that any patients should be instructed to sleep with the correct pillow and sleeping posture as part of their lifestyle guidance.

2.3.2 The Pillow Clinic: Procedures in the First Day

The procedures for a patient visiting the Pillow Clinic on the first day are summarized in Fig. 2.10. The first step is to complete a medical questionnaire by the patient. Then the questionnaire is checked by a nursing assistant to ensure whether it contains all the necessary information for diagnosis, and if not, additional interviews are performed and the information is inputted into the electronic medical record. At this point, difference of the Pillow Clinic from other general outpatient clinics is that we ask detailed information about the patient's living and sleeping environments, particularly the information about the bedding (pillow, mattress/futon, comforter, pajamas, bed partner, etc.). Additional information is also obtained on the sleep disorders and its past treatment and medication histories. Based on the information, the physician conducts palpation and some tests, to instruct any necessary image diagnosis. Using the findings of image diagnosis, a comprehensive diagnosis is made and the physician feedbacks to the patient on the diagnosis, the disease conditions, the treatment plan, then hears patient's wishes, obtain patient's consent, and then the treatment is initiated. At this time, if there are any problems with the patient's sleep environment and posture, we point out it and instruct how to correct them. For example, if the patient's bedding or bed is inappropriate, we will explain the points and materials to be changed, and for the pillow, we will give specific instructions on the materials and methods of making a handmade pillow. Table 2.2 summarizes the typical problems on bedding and the points of instruction

Interview
- Symptoms, disease history.
- Living environment, sleeping environment and bedding information (pillow, mattress, comforter), pyjamas, bed partner, etc.

Exami-nation
- palpation
- Tests for diagnosis

Labo. tests
- X-ray examination
- Magnetic Resonance Imaging (MRI)
- Blood tests, etc.

Diagnosis
- Definitive diagnosis and description of the condition

Therapy
- Treatment planning - medication, injections, rehabilitation, lifestyle guidance, especially posture guidance, etc.

Daytime postural guidance: standing, sitting, walking, etc.
Nighttime postural guidance: bedding guidance for correct sleeping posture

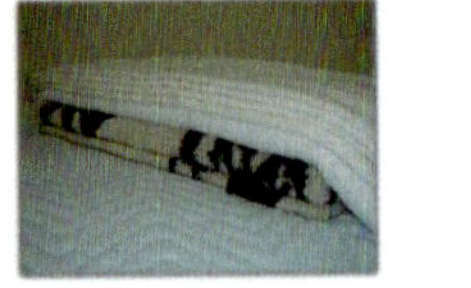

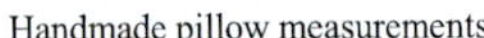

Handmade pillow measurements

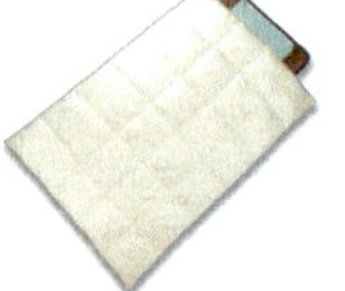

Guidance for beddings

Fig. 2.10 Procedures of the first day in pillow clinic

Table 2.2 Typical bedding problems and guidance points

Beddings	Factor	Information	Guidance points
Bed, futon, mattress	Materials	Down, wool, cotton, polyester fiber, buckwheat hulls, plastic chips, cypress chips, various types of polyurethane foam (low rebound, high resilience), latex, air fiber, etc.	Materials that sink or warp in the hips or back during sleep are problematic
	Years of use		Maintenance and replacement period is around 6 years for futons and 12 years for mattresses (depending on the material, etc.)
	Purchase method	Shop, online shopping, online retailing	Mattresses are tools used in contact with the body and should be purchased after experiencing them
	Maintenance	Frequency of changing backs and fronts, or changing tops and bottoms	Varies according to material, but should be used back to front or head and foot interchangeably to prevent deterioration
	Multiple use	Use of same or different materials in layers	Note that body support changes depending on the material and number of layers
	Usage status		If you experience spinal or back problems from the moment you wake up, your mattress may be unsuitable
Pillow	Materials	Down, wool, cotton, polyester fiber, buckwheat hulls, plastic chips, cypress chips, various types of polyurethane foam (low resilience, high elasticity), latex, air fiber, etc.	Materials that change the height of the pillow during sleep are problematic
	Years of use		The fit of the pillow to the body should be reviewed every two years
	Purchase Method	Shop, online shopping, online retailing	Pillows are tools used in contact with the body and should be purchased after experiencing them
	Maintenance	Self-adjustment (height and content)	Pillow height needs to be fine-tuned to the millimeter. So a commercial pillow is unlikely to fit and needs to be adjusted
	Multiple use	Stacking of two or more pillows	Multiple pillows collapse during sleep. Only one pillow with adjusted height should be used
	Usage status	defects (especially on awakening, if the pillow has not moved away from under the head)	If you feel more neck and shoulder problems from the moment you wake up, it is possible that your pillow is not suitable

2.3.3 Diseases for Pillow Prescription

Since the Pillow Clinic was opened in 2002, about 60% and 30% of the patients came to the clinic complaining of shoulder stiffness and of back pain, respectively. Many of the shoulder stiffness were chronic and intractable, and some of the patients complained that they had been suffering for about 30 years. Large number of the patients complained of not only shoulder stiffness but also many other physical symptoms and had been repeatedly doctor-shopping many times with main complaint of shoulder stiffness.

The diseases for the pillow therapy are mainly divided into two categories (Table 2.3): one is symptoms and diseases that have been validated at the clinical research level. Another is those that have not yet been validated at the clinical research level, but have been judged to be empirically effective on a clinical experience basis. How much physicians place importance on evidence when selecting a treatment depends on the physician and the nature of the treatment. Of course, treatments with sufficient evidence should be selected. However, even if any evidence for a particular symptom or disease is not clearly stated, if it is safe and the patient is fully informed and consents, it may be worth a try. With this in mind, we have presented the two categories.

Pillow adjustment is not only for primary shoulder stiffness, but also for physical symptoms such as headache, dizziness, and insomnia, caused by cervical spine disease, lumbar spine disease, shoulder joint disease, and so on. It is applicable to both acute and chronic symptoms. For example, if cervical rest can be taken as early as possible in the acute phase of a cervical sprain using the optimal pillow, the transition to the chronic phase is prevented in some cases. The optimal pillow can also relieve pains in acute phase of periarthritis of the shoulder joint or calcific rotator cuff tendonitis. In turning over or lateral position, the pillow may reduce the load on the shoulder joint and relieve increased intra-articular pressure. Interestingly, even in traumatic injuries such as rib fractures, an appropriately adjusted pillow may reduce the load on the fracture during

Table 2.3 Indications for pillow guidance

Diseases for which evidence has been proven by our clinical research	Diseases for which efficacy has been determined by our experience
• Shoulder stiffness (including refractory shoulder stiffness) • Osteoarthritis of the cervical spine • Cervical disc herniation • Cervical spondylotic radiculopathy • Tension-type headache • Rheumatoid arthritis • Abnormal postures (kyphosis, scoliosis) • Chronic pain (chronic neck pain) • Somatic symptoms • Sleep apnea syndrome (mild/moderate)	• Cervical spinal canal stenosis • Whiplash injury • Dropped head syndrome • Shoulder-arm syndrome • Periarthritis of shoulder (nocturnal pain) • Knee osteoarthritis (nocturnal pain) • Low back pain (nocturnal pain) • Rib fracture (nocturnal pain) • Pediatric neck pain, stiff shoulders, headache • Temporomandibular joint disorder • Snoring

nighttime turning over, thereby reducing pain. Some patients who visited us in the chronic phase of their disease showed improvement in a relatively short period after pillow adjustment. Based on a 6-year follow-up of a patient with rheumatoid arthritis, it was suggested that repeated pillow adjustment therapy improves ankylosis into a good supine cervical spine alignment, and therefore we are actively incorporating this therapy into our daily life guidance for patients. For patients with postural abnormalities, especially in cases of kyphosis or scoliosis, who complain of pain during sleep and upon awakening, pain management through nocturnal postural guidance is beneficial. In terms of nocturnal pain, those caused by periarthritis of the shoulder, osteoarthritis of the knee, and low back pain have been effectively improved. However, in some cases, it is difficult to completely resolve daytime pain or improve limitations of motion using the pillow. Bedding adjustments should first be applied for the reduction of during sleeping and upon waking pains.

In addition, it is also indicated as an adjunctive therapy for other medical conditions, such as snoring in otolaryngology, moderate cases of sleep apnea syndrome (excluding severe cases with continuous positive airway pressure (CPAP) therapy), and chronic pain, tension-type headache, and temporomandibular joint disorder, which are typical symptoms of functional somatic syndrome (FSS) in internal medicine.

2.3.4 Pillow Consultation

The benefit of pillow therapy is the ability to provide effective and safe treatment with a low cost for chronic neck pain, shoulder stiffness, and any pains and complaints occurring during sleep that are intractable and no optimal treatment.

Pillow adjustment does not complete only once. If symptoms flare up after a period of improvement, the patient should be asked again about the pillow and bedding situation. This means to confirm whether the pillow has not been compressed or the patient's physique has not changed and the previously adjusted pillow is still suitable. As mentioned in the definition of the Pillow Clinic, "good sleep" is an underlying fundamental infrastructure for recovering patient's physical condition. That is why instructors must repeatedly guide and check patients until they are able to manage their own bedding environment. In practice, there are two categories of instructors in hospitals and clinics.

2.3.4.1 In Case a Nurse or Nursing Assistant Instructs Pillow Adjustments

In preparation of the treatment plan and if the physician determines that daytime and nighttime postural guidance is necessary among the daily lifestyle guidance (including diet, exercise, and posture guidance), the physician informs the nurse or nursing assistant accordingly. Pillow adjustment is included in nighttime postural guidance as it is a factor that determines sleep posture

2.3.4.2 In Case a Physical Therapist Instructs the Pillow Adjustments

As in the case of nurses, when a physician determines that the patient needs to adjust his or her sleeping posture, the physician informs the physical therapist accordingly.

Patients who are eligible for compensating the musculoskeletal rehabilitation fee are those with chronic musculoskeletal disorders that have resulted in a certain degree of decline in motor function and daily living ability. For example, patients with osteoarthritis, cervical or lumbar disc disease, degenerative joint disease, inflammatory disease of joints, joint contracture, or musculoskeletal instability.

Here is a specific case: a 60-year-old woman with cervical spondylotic radiculopathy. Her chief complaint is cervical pain, right upper extremity pain, and numbness in her right hand from the time she wakes up. Her symptoms are mild during the day and at work, but worsen when she sleeps or wakes up, and a thorough MRI examination revealed a cervical disc herniation. In response, the physician prescribes musculoskeletal rehabilitation to instruct her to manage the posture both during the day and at night while sleeping to avoid pains. The diagnosis is cervical spondylotic radiculopathy, and the rehabilitation instructions include "improve cervical posture during the day and at bedtime and to instruct pillow adjustment." The short-term treatment goals are "improvement of neck pain and other symptoms while sleeping and awakening" and "acquisition of turning movements while sleeping"; the specific methods are " adjustment of bedding environment and pillow" and "turning movement training." The physical therapist will point out problems with the patient's current pillow, instruct the patient on how to adjust the pillow correctly, and explain the specific materials and how to make the handmade pillow. It is important to guide the patient to adjust their pillow by themselves at home. At a later date, the patient brings his/her own pillow from home and the physical therapist checks for its fitness. The physical therapist places the patient in bed and checks a supine position, lateral position, and turning over to determine the optimal pillow height. The patient must readjust as his or her physique changes and posture ages (e.g., kyphosis). During the consultation, the physician assesses the patient's pillow fitness and instructs the physiotherapist to readjust the pillow if the patient's once-improved symptoms flare up.

References

1. OECD. Health spending (indicator). Paris: OECD; 2022. https://doi.org/10.1787/8643de7e-en. Accessed 26 May 2022.
2. Jackson R. The cervical syndrome. 2nd ed. Springfield, IL: Charles C. Thomas; 1958. p. 157–61.
3. Jackson R. The cervical syndrome. 4th ed. Springfield, IL: Charles C. Thomas; 1977. p. 310–5.
4. Cervipillo®. The 1967 National Assembly of the American orthotic and prosthetic association, the orthopedic and prosthetic appliance journal. Washington, DC: American Orthotic and Prosthetic Association; 1967. p. 173.
5. Jackson R. The classic: the cervical syndrome. 1949. Clin Orthop Relat Res. 2010;468(7):1739–45. https://doi.org/10.1007/s11999-010-1278-8. PMID: 20177837; PMCID: PMC2881998.

6. Ren S, Wong DW-C, Yang H, Zhou Y, Lin J, Zhang M. Effect of pillow height on the biomechanics of the head-neck complex: investigation of the cranio-cervical pressure and cervical spine alignment. PeerJ. 2016;4:e2397. https://doi.org/10.7717/peerj.2397.
7. Gordon SJ, Trott P, Grimmer KA. Waking cervical pain and stiffness, headache, scapular or arm pain: gender and age effects. Aust J Physiother. 2002;48(1):9–15. https://doi.org/10.1016/s0004-9514(14)60277-4.
8. Erfanian P, Hagino CC, Guerriero RC. A preliminary study assessing adverse effects of a semi-customized cervical pillow on asymptomatic adults. J Can Chiropr Assoc. 1998;42(3):156–62.
9. Lin X-Y, Wu F-G. Pillow shape design to enhance the sleep quality of middle-aged groups. Proc Manuf. 2015;3:4429–35.
10. Jeon MY, Jeong HC, Lee SW, Choi W, Park JH, Tak SJ, et al. Improving the quality of sleep with an optimal pillow: a randomized, comparative study. Tohoku J Exp Med. 2014;233(3):183–8.
11. Lee JH, Shin J-S, Yoo H-K, Lee J, Lee YJ, Kim M-R, et al. Short-term effects of a functional cervical pillow on inpatients with neck discomfort: a randomized controlled trial. Int J Clin Exp Med. 2016;9(6):11397–408.
12. Yim JE. Optimal pillow conditions for high-quality sleep: a theoretical review. Indian J Sci Technol. 2015;8(S5):135–9.
13. Gordon SJ, Grimmer-Somers KA, Trott PH. A randomized, comparative trial: does pillow type alter cervico-thoracic spinal posture when side lying? J Multidiscip Healthc. 2011;4:321–7.
14. Gordon SJ, Grimmer-Somers K, Trott P. Pillow use: the behaviour of cervical pain, sleep quality and pillow comfort in side sleepers. Man Ther. 2009;14(6):671–8.
15. Gordon SJ, Grimmer-Somers KA, Trott PH. Pillow use: the behavior of cervical stiffness, headache and scapular/arm pain. J Pain Res. 2010;3:137–45.
16. Lavin RA, Pappagallo M, Kuhlemeier KV. Cervical pain: a comparison of three pillows. Arch Phys Med Rehabil. 1997;78(2):193–8. https://doi.org/10.1016/s0003-9993(97)90263-x.
17. Gordon SJ, Grimmer-Somers K. Your pillow may not guarantee a good night's sleep or symptom-free waking. Physiother Can. 2011;63(2):183–90.
18. Erfanian P, Tenzif S, Guerriero RC. Assessing effects of a semi-customized experimental cervical pillow on symptomatic adults with chronic neck pain with and without headache. J Can Chiropr Assoc. 2004;48(1):20–8.
19. Fazli F, Farahmand B, Azadinia F, Amiri A. A preliminary study: the effect of ergonomic latex pillow on pain and disability in patients with cervical spondylosis. Med J Islam Repub Iran. 2018;32:81. https://doi.org/10.14196/mjiri.32.81.
20. Gross AR, Kaplan F, Huang S, Khan M, Santaguida PL, Carlesso LC, et al. Psychological care, patient education, orthotics, ergonomics and prevention strategies for neck pain: an systematic overview update as part of the icon§ project. Open Orthop J. 2013;7:530–61. https://doi.org/10.2174/1874325001307010530.
21. Hurwitz EL, Carragee EJ, van der Velde G, Carroll LJ, Nordin M, Guzman J, et al. Treatment of neck pain: noninvasive interventions. Results of the bone and joint decade 2000–2010 task force on neck pain and its associated disorders. Eur Spine J. 2008;17(Suppl 1):123–52. https://doi.org/10.1007/s00586-008-0631-z.
22. Gordon SJ, Grimmer KA, Buttner P. Pillow preferences of people with neck pain and known spinal degeneration: a pilot randomized controlled trial. Eur J Phys Rehabil Med. 2019;55(6):783–91. https://doi.org/10.23736/S1973-9087.19.05263-8.
23. Radwan A, Ashton N, Gates T, Kilmer A, Van Fleet M. Effect of different pillow designs on promoting sleep comfort, quality, & spinal alignment: a systematic review. Eur J Integr Med. 2021;42:101269. https://doi.org/10.1016/j.eujim.2020.101269.
24. Wang J-C, Chan R-C, Wu H-L, Lai C-J. Effect of pillow size preference on extensor digitorum communis muscle strength and electromyographic activity during maximal contraction in healthy individuals: a pilot study. J Chin Med Assoc. 2015;78(3):182–7. https://doi.org/10.1016/j.jcma.2014.09.005. Epub 2014 Oct 30.
25. Shields N, Capper J, Polak T, Taylor N. Are cervical pillows effective in reducing neck pain? N Z J Physiother. 2006;34(1):3–9.

26. Pang JCY, Tsang SMH, Fu ACL. The effects of pillow designs on neck pain, waking symptoms, neck disability, sleep quality and spinal alignment in adults: a systematic review and meta-analysis. Clin Biomech. 2021;85:105353. https://doi.org/10.1016/j.clinbiomech.2021.105353.
27. Takano J. A pillow that can make you healthy and sleep well. 2018. http://www.pyroenergen.com/articles08/healthy-pillow.htm. Accessed 10 Apr 2022.
28. Cai D, Chen H-L. Ergonomic approach for pillow concept design. Appl Ergon. 2016;52:142–50.
29. Liu S-F, Lee Y-L, Liang J-C. Shape design of an optimal comfortable pillow based on the analytic hierarchy process method. J Chiropr Med. 2011;10(4):229–39. https://doi.org/10.1016/j.jcm.2011.04.002. PMID: 22654680; PMCID: PMC3315854.
30. Her J-G, Ko D-H, Woo J-H, Choi Y-E. Development and comparative evaluation of new shapes of pillows. J Phys Ther Sci. 2014;26(3):377–80. https://doi.org/10.1589/jpts.26.377. Epub 2014 Mar 25. PMID: 24707087; PMCID: PMC3976006.
31. Sacco ICN, Pereira ILR, Dinato RC, Silva VC, Friso B, Viterbo SF. The effect of pillow height on muscle activity of the neck and mid-upper back and patient perception of comfort. J Manipulative Physiol Ther. 2015;38(6):375–81. https://doi.org/10.1016/j.jmpt.2015.06.012. Epub 2015 Jul 21.
32. Kim HC, Jun HS, Kim JH, Ahn JH, Chang IB, Song JH, et al. The effect of different pillow heights on the parameters of cervicothoracic spine segments. Korean J Spine. 2015;12(3):135–8. https://doi.org/10.14245/kjs.2015.12.3.135. Epub 2015 Sep 30.
33. Son J, Jung S, Song H, Kim J, Bang S, Bahn S. A survey of Koreans on sleep habits and sleeping symptoms relating to pillow comfort and support. Int J Environ Res Public Health. 2020;17(1):302. https://doi.org/10.3390/ijerph17010302.

3 Case Reports

Abstract

In this chapter, we report some impressive patients encountered in our daily practices in the Pillow Clinic. They are the patients who have improved significantly by the pillow therapy. Their background characteristics, pre-treatment pillows, medical interviews, findings of imaging, optimal pillow heights, and clinical courses after adjusted pillow use are presented. These reports help you to imagine more easily the effects of the pillow therapy to be conducted by yourself.

Keywords

Cervical spine disorders · Neck and shoulder stiffness · Headache · Dizziness · Dropped head syndrome · Sleep disorders

Data 3.1 presents several cases in adults in which symptoms improved with the use of an optimal pillow.

Cervical disc herniation, Cervical spondylosis, Cervical spondylotic radiculopathy, Central spinal cord injury, Ossification of the cervical longitudinal ligament (OPLL), Dropped head syndrome, Ankylosing spondylitis, Shoulder stiffness, Headache, Dizziness, Periarthritis of the shoulder joint, Rheumatoid arthritis, High dislocation of the hip joint, Lumbar osteoarthritis, Sciatica, Postural abnormalities (kyphosis, lordosis, scoliosis, straight neck), Snoring, Sleep apnea syndrome (SAS), Insomnia, Sleep on one's neck wrong, Sleep disorders, Fibromyalgia, Parkinson's disease, etc.

Supplementary Information The online version contains supplementary material available at https://doi.org/10.1007/978-981-99-0463-1_3.

S. Yamada, *Orthopaedic Pillow*, https://doi.org/10.1007/978-981-99-0463-1_3

Basic Knowledge About Pillows

4

Abstract

This chapter outlines problems with the materials, shapes, sizes, and choices of pillows available in the market around 2020. In Japan, Korea, Europe, and the USA, mainly used pillows are the conventional ordinary pillows made by cotton or down and the recently increasing contour pillows. Our internet survey in 2020 found a discrepancy between the pillows and sleep requirements that pillow users consider important and the characteristics of the pillows they actually use. These results suggest that pillow users have no clear criteria for selecting a pillow. We introduce three major requirements for pillows that have been proposed since 2002. These are the basic requirements for adjusting a pillow to fit each individual's skeletal structure, regardless of race or preference. The role of the pillow is to support the vital physiological phenomenon of turning over during sleeping time. The Set-up for Spinal Sleep method (SSS method) is a method for determining the pillow height to adjust an individual in all sleep positions including supine and lateral positions and turning over. The important points and specific steps of this method are explained.

Keywords

Commercially available pillows · Ordinary pillow · Contour pillow · Pillow requirements · Set-up for spinal sleep method (SSS method) · Turning over

4.1 Materials, Shapes, and Sizes of Commercially Available Pillows, and Their Selection and Problems

In Japan, marketed pillows are made by so many kinds of materials that are impossible to count. They include down, feather, polyester, cotton, wool, low resilience urethane, high elasticity urethane, latex, buckwheat hull, cypress, red beans, plastic

S. Yamada, *Orthopaedic Pillow*, https://doi.org/10.1007/978-981-99-0463-1_4

chips, microbeads, and so on. In recent years, Artificial Intelligence (AI) or sensors have also been built into pillows to monitor the condition of brain and body during sleep. Some pillows are as large as from head to shoulder, or long enough to be used by two or more people. The shapes of pillows are also becoming more complex, such as donut-shaped, contour vertically or horizontally, or ones divided into five or six parts filled with different materials. The variety of pillows in Japan is outstanding compared to other countries. In Japan, pillow specialty stores or department stores having pillow corners have appeared since around 2000, and pillow sales have become a trend. Many patients in the Pillow Clinic say, "There are so many kinds of pillow and materials on the market, I don't know which the pillow fits the best." I think this statement is to the point.

A similar phenomenon may also be seen in South Korea, Japan's neighboring country. In 2020, South Korean researchers Juhyun Son et al. [1] researched habits and symptoms of sleep related to pillow comfort and support in Koreans. In the research, they systematically reviewed preceding reported studies on pillow and collected information on more than 200 of commercially available pillows, then categorized them into six types according to shape and contour, and asked participants which type they used. The six pillow types were: pillows of regular-type, contour-type, peanut-shaped, functional A-type, functional B-type, and others (Wooden pillow, etc.). These are products that are commonly also seen in Japan in recent years and can be easily purchased online. Results showed that although 54% of subjects used regular-type pillows, they had lower satisfactions on multiple factors of comfort and support (supportive, amenity, and fitness of pillow height and shape) compared to participants using functional-type pillows.

Whenever I traveled to the USA in recent years, I actually visited and investigated pillow retailers. In both New York and Silicon Valley, pillow and bedding specialty stores were lined with around $100 of pillows made by latex, low rebound urethane, or high elastic urethane, while shopping centers were piled with polyester or cotton ordinary pillows costing around $10. Especially in the USA, I frequently heard the talking, "Pillows are used only when we are lying on the side, and don't use it on the upward."

In 2020, we conducted an online survey of 124 people aged 19–78 years (mean age 38.6 years) from 11 countries around the world to investigate what type of pillow they use and their awareness toward pillows using a questionnaire (Fig. 4.1). The most commonly used type of pillow was a cotton pillow or ordinary pillow (74.8%), followed by a contour pillow (14.6%) and others (Fig. 4.2). We confirmed that although pillows with various materials and shapes have been introduced, the conventional cotton pillow is still overwhelmingly the mainstream. Interestingly, there was a discrepancy between the answers in awareness survey, with 79% of respondents saying that they need to turn over during sleep, and 37% believing that it is easier to turn over when using a pillow of the right height, and actual situation with around 80% of respondents still use soft, fluffy, easily height-changeable cotton pillows. This fact suggests the issue that pillow users have no criteria for choosing a pillow. This is a study accepted for the 13th annual community college Honor Research Symposium held at the University of California, Berkeley in 2020.

Fig. 4.1 Internet survey on pillows in 2020 ($N = 124$)

		(Number of people)
1.	U.S.A	62
2.	Philippines	31
3.	Japan	16
4.	U.K.	4
5.	France, Australia, Canada, Argenitina	2 each
6.	Tunisia, Iceland, Singapore	1 each

Share rates of pillows used in the world

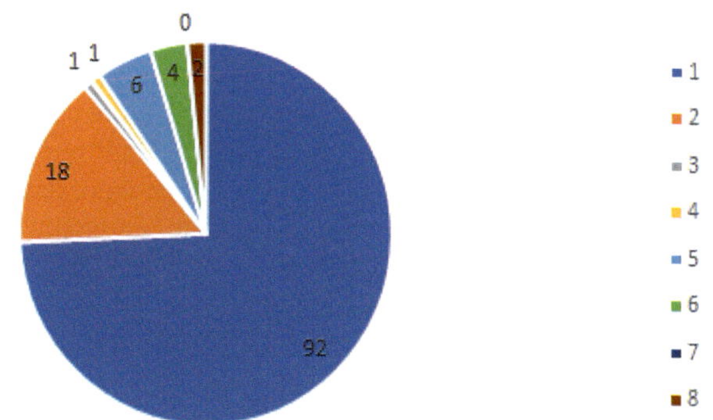

Pillow Types

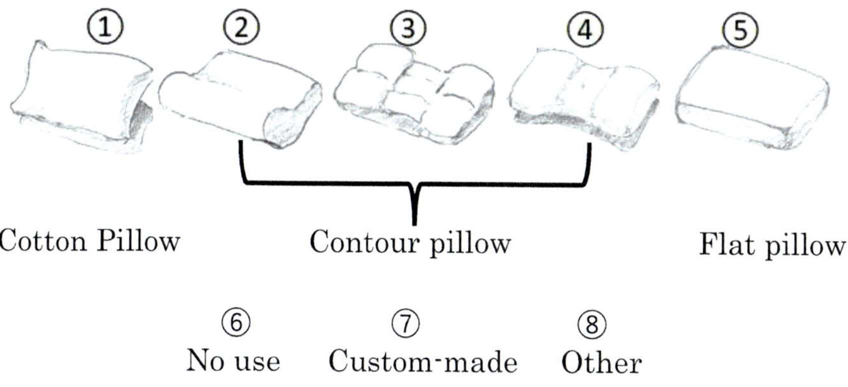

Fig. 4.2 Types of pillows used in the world. No. 1, cotton pillow; No. 2, contour pillow

4.2 Three Major Requirements for an Optimal Pillow

The three major requirements for an optimal pillow, in my opinion, are as follows. The first is optimal height that is adjusted to individual physique. Determine the single height that is suitable for both supine and lateral sleeping positions. The second is to determine proper firmness that does not sink more than 5 mm all-night. The third is flat surface to turn over easily. In addition, it is needed to readjust depending on changes in physique or aging (Fig. 4.3).

I believe that the most important pillow requirement is height, and the importance of pillow height has been discussed in the world in recent years. Jia-Xing Lei et al. [2] reviewed the current trends, research methodologies, and determinants of pillow height evaluation, summarizing the evidence published from 1997 to 2021. They concluded that the suggested range for achieving optimal cervical spine alignment, appropriate pressure distribution, and minimal muscle activity during sleep cannot yet be identified. In addition, they said that there remain no firm conclusions about the optimal pillow height for the supine and lateral positions. Their fundamental idea is that the optimal pillow height should maintain the physiological curvature of the cervical spine during sleep.

We cannot say that we have sufficient scientific evidence to say whether our idea of pillow adjustment is correct. However, we successfully developed an algorithm based on large amount of data on pillow heights showing clinical efficacy and concluded no need to curvature the cervical spine alignment during sleep.

Let's describe the actual orthopedic pillow we use in our research in detail. The size is 30 cm (length) × 60 cm (width) × adjustable (height) and is made by laminate sheets of urethane or polyethylene for precise adjustment of height at a pitch of 5 mm. Figure 4.4 shows an example of the orthopedic pillow, a combination of pillow materials and height-adjusting sheets, and Table 4.1. shows the optimal pillow heights based on body height/weight and age in Japanese population. These are only a guide and need to be adjusted more strictly according to the individual physique.

Fig. 4.3 Three major requirements for an optimal pillow

Three major pillow requirements

1. Optimal height
   It is adjusted to individual physique

2. Proper Firmness
   It does not sink more than 5 mm

3. Flat Surface
   It is easy to turn over in sleep

And Re-adjustment
(to accommodate changes in body physique and aging)

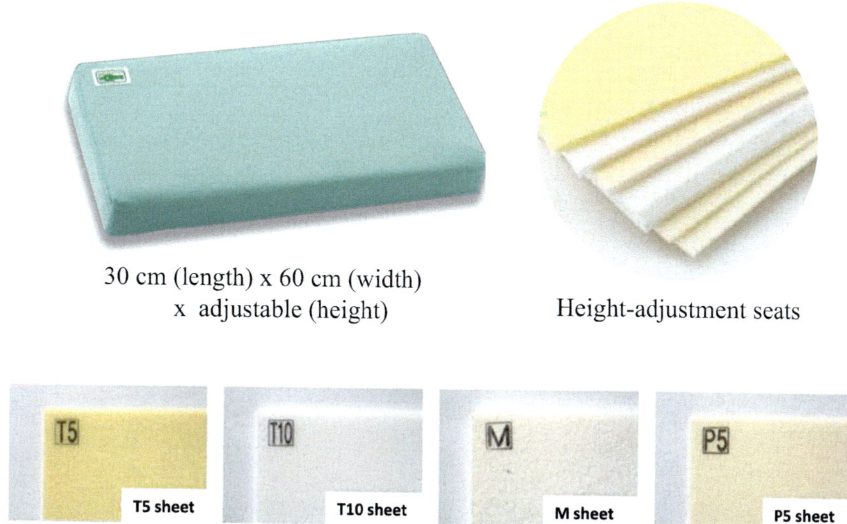

T5: 5 mm-thick sheet of low resilience urethane
T10: 10 mm-thick sheet of low resilience urethane
M: 20 mm or 35 mm-thick sheets of mixed urethane
P5: 5 mm-thick sheet of polyethylene

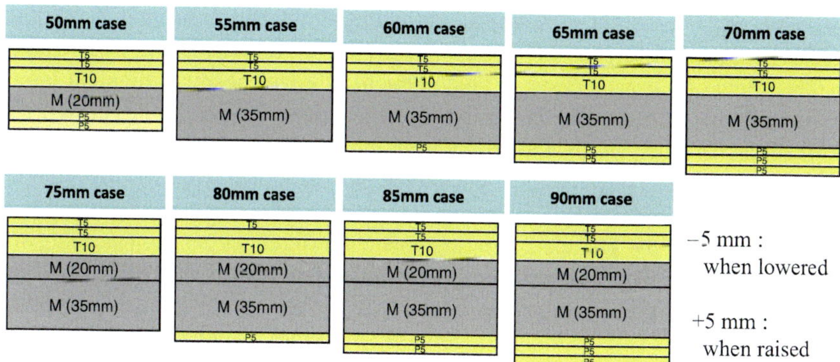

Fig. 4.4 Examples of the orthopaedic pillow (made by height-adjusting sheets)

Conversely, in the Pillow Clinic, patients are allowed to bring their own materials to create handmade pillows. The best materials are a Japanese entrance mat (about 50 cm wide × 90 cm long × 1 cm thick) and a large towelket (a blanket made of toweling), both of moderately stiff materials. If these are layered, it can substitute for the orthopedic pillow. The following video explains the method to make the handmade pillow by the SSS Method. (Video File 2, https://www.youtube.com/watch?v=iRZ0Th73kNk&t=70s).

Table 4.1 Example of optimal pillow height based on body height/weight and age (in Japanese population)

Gender	Height (cm)	Weight (kg)	Pillow height (mm)
Pillow height by height and weight for people in their 30s			
Female	150	45	55
	158	54	60
	165	60	65
Male	160	60	70
	171	69	75
	180	75	80
Pillow height by height and weight for people in their 60s			
Female	150	45	60
	158	54	65
	165	60	70
Male	160	60	75
	171	69	80
	180	75	85

4.3 The Role of the Pillows

Many people, including medical professionals, think that a pillow is an item that determines the position of the head and the angle of the cervical spine. However, after adjusting the height of more than 60,000 pillows and observing the turning over of people of different body sizes and ages in children and elderly, we realized that the effect of pillow is never limited to the head, cervical spine, shoulder joints, and other parts of the upper body, but also the thoracolumbar spine, pelvis, and lower limbs. In other words, the pillow is an indispensable gear, body tool, during sleep to support "the physiological phenomenon of turn over, which is essential for maintaining life." In the field of ergonomics, "body tool" is an equipment that is in contact with the body. There are two fundamental differences between sleeping and waking postures. When we are awake, our muscles support our skeletal balance and maintain good posture. During sleep, however, as we are not conscious, we need the suitable bedding to help us maintain good sleep posture. Another is with regard to dynamic movement. While awake, we are capable of all kinds of skillful movements under conscious awareness. During sleep, we cannot be perfectly static because we are living things, so we must keep moving. That is why we are turning over. However, since sleep is originally for preserving physical strength and recovering tired body tissues, we want to perform turning over movements efficiently with minimum energy. Figure 4.5 shows the center axis of rotation for turning over on an optimal pillow.

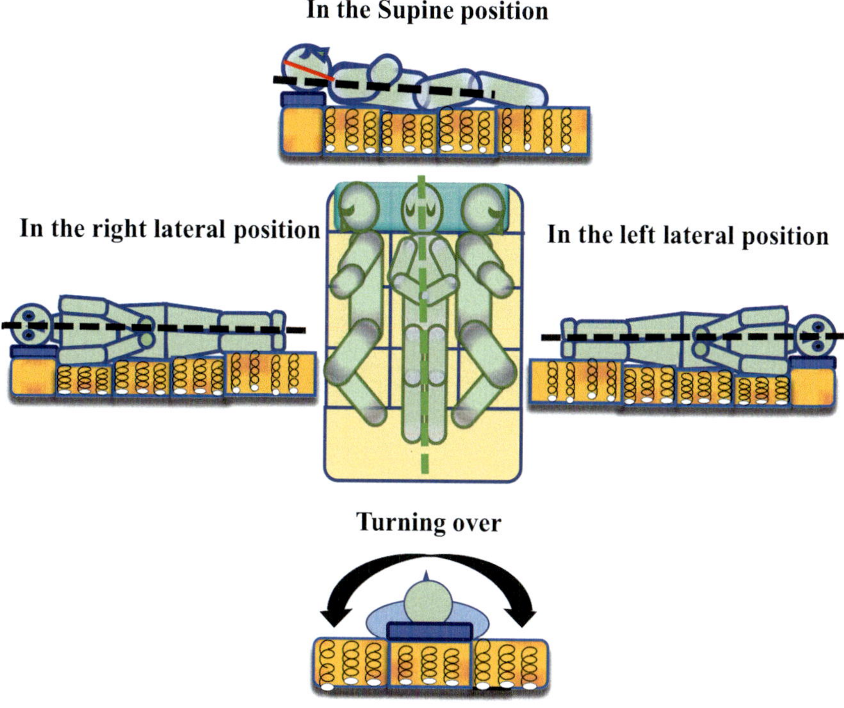

Fig. 4.5 Center axis of rotation for turning over when using the optimal pillow

4.4 Set-Up for Spinal Sleep (SSS) Method

The SSS method of pillow adjustment consists of three steps (Fig. 4.6). While it is more accurate if confirmed by X-ray or MRI, in the outpatient clinic, the medical professional macroscopically check it in patient's body surface.

Step 1: The patient is supine position with upper and lower limbs in extension and relaxation. The examiner adjusts the height of the pillow by changing the height in 5-mm increments toward the supine cervical tilt angle of approximately 15°, asking the subject how much comfortable for feelings on breath at both exhalations and inhalations, the occipital area, and muscle tension in the posterior neck.

Step 2: Check at the left and right side in the lateral positions. First, in the supine position, the patient is placed in the " the turn over position" with both forearms crossed over the anterior chest, the right hand touching the left clavicle and the left hand touching the right clavicle, both hip joints flexed to approximately 60°, and both knees flexed to around 100°. Second, rotate to the right and left to lie on lateral

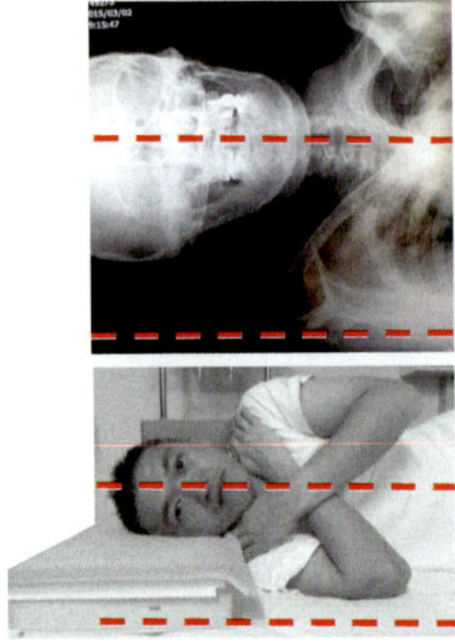

1st step: In lateral position

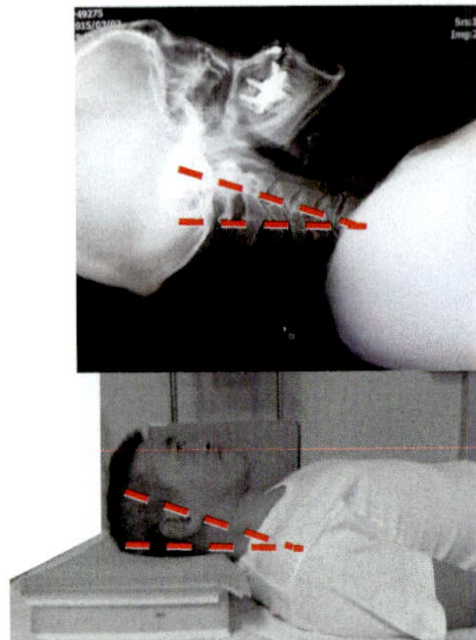

2nd step: In supine position

Set up for Spinal Sleep method (SSS method) is a method adjusting the height of -pillow for each person.

1st step: In the lateral position, the pillow height is adjusted so that the axis of head and trunk of the subject is aligned in parallel with the bed surface.

2nd step: In the supine position, the cervical spine is held at an angle of approximately 15 degrees anterior tilt from the bed surface.

3rd step: In the dynamic motion, we check how smoothly the subject is able to turn over according to the different height of pillow, adjusting increments and decrements of 5mm.

Finally, the pillow height that enables the subject to turn over most smoothly is the optimal adjusted pillow.

Fig. 4.6 Set up for Spinal Sleep Method (SSS Method) (JP2004209099A)

positions. The height is adjusted so that the bed surface is parallel to the centerline of the head and neck that passes through the forehead, nose, chin, and sternum. It is also helpful to ask questions of the subject on tensions in the sternocleidomastoid and levator scapulae muscles. If the optimal height is unequal for the left and right sides, determine the optimal height by observing the patient turning over described in the next step.

Step 3: Check the smoothness of turning over. In the supine position, let the patient at the turn over position and rotate two or three times to the left or right and then compare the smoothness of the turn over. Macroscopic smoothness is defined as synchronized rotation of the head, chest, and pelvis with respect to the central axis. Conversely, the un-smoothness is a condition in which misalignment is generated in each part of movement. When evaluates using the acromion of the scapula and the greater trochanter of the femur as indicators, awkward movements are observed, such as a delay in one or the other, or a great deal of force or recoil on a part of the body to compensate with muscle power against the delay. The optimal pillow height is the one that allows the patient to turn over most smoothly.

A handmade pillow made by folded and laminated materials brought with the patient can be substituted. Photographs and X-ray images of the cervical spine alignment at different pillow heights are shown in Fig. 4.7. The subject is the author at 38 years old, about 20 years ago. At that time, my optimal pillow height was 50 mm. At the lateral position with that height, the axis of the head and neck passing through the forehead, nose, chin, and sternum was aligned in parallel with the bed surface. In the supine position, the cervical tilt angle was approximately 15°, which made turning over the most smoothly. Twenty years have passed since then, and the optimal height of the author's pillow is currently 65 mm, which is higher than before. This was thought to be due to an increase in body weight of 5 kg and a decrease in flexibility of the bone joints with aging.

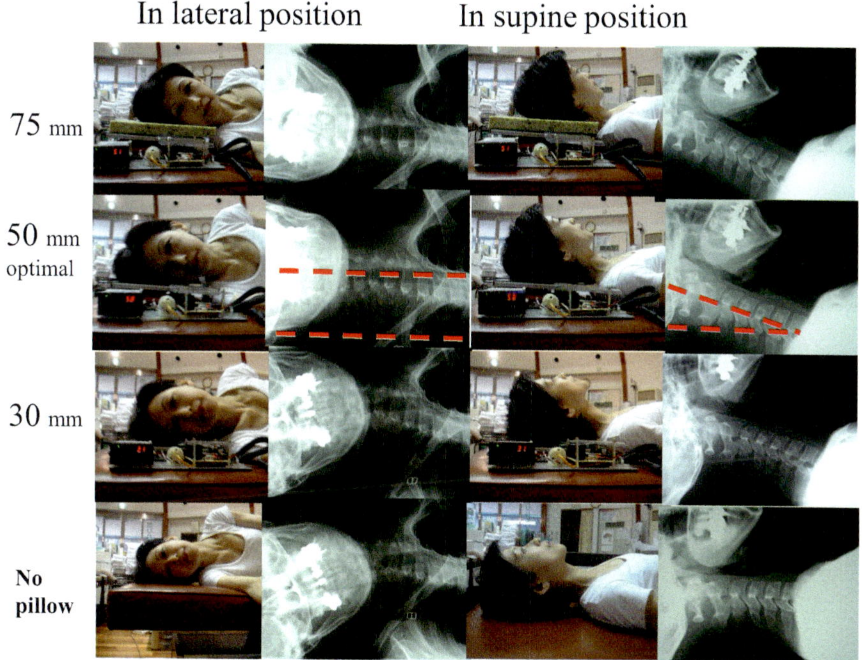

At an optimal pillow height (50 mm), Cervical alignment is;

In the lateral position, the axis of head and trunk is aligned in parallel with the bed surface.

In the supine position, the cervical tilt angle is approximately 15° .

Fig. 4.7 Pillow height and cervical spine alignment

References

1. Son J, Jung S, Song H, Kim J, Bang S, Bahn S. A survey of Koreans on sleep habits and sleeping symptoms relating to pillow comfort and support. Int J Environ Res Public Health. 2020;17(1):302. https://doi.org/10.3390/ijerph17010302.
2. Lei J-X, Yang P-F, Yang A-L, Gong Y-F, Shang P, Yuan X-C. Ergonomic consideration in pillow height determinants and evaluation. Healthcare (Basel). 2021;9(10):1333. https://doi.org/10.3390/healthcare9101333.

5 Basic Research on Pillows

Abstract

In this chapter, we introduce our basic and clinical researches on pillow to determine the optimal pillow using the Set-up for Spinal Sleep Method (the SSS Method) described in Sect. 4.4. First, we examined a relationship between the optimal pillows and body sizes, i.e., height, weight, and other physical characteristics. By using X-ray and MRI, the cervical spine alignments in the optimal pillow revealed a universal cervical spine angle. Second, the motion capture system was used to analyze not only the static but also the dynamic postures of the human body, such as turning over in bed. Video analysis of all-night turning overs was performed, and new knowledge about turning over was obtained. Third, relation between pillows and straight neck, which is considered to be a cervical spine malposition, is examined. We also studied pillow adjustment for special diseases such as rheumatoid arthritis, kyphosis, trauma (cervical sprain), and sleep apnea syndrome. Finally, we analyzed images of the pillows of 0-year-old newborns and children and obtained interesting findings.

Keywords

Straight neck · Rheumatoid Arthritis · Kyphosis · Whiplash injury · Sleep apnea syndrome · Infant and children

---

Supplementary Information The online version contains supplementary material available at https://doi.org/10.1007/978-981-99-0463-1_5.

S. Yamada, *Orthopaedic Pillow*, https://doi.org/10.1007/978-981-99-0463-1_5

Scientific and empirical validations are essential as long as the pillow adjustment is recommended to patients at a therapeutic level. Conversely, however, trusting evidence only from articles published in high impact factor journals and applying them to daily practice may lead to overlook beneficial treatments that have not yet scientifically verified. We strongly encourage readers to use our validated evidence, the pillow therapy, demonstrated here in your clinical practice, experience its efficacy, and gradually expand the application range and treatment targets (Fig. 5.1).

In Chap. 1, we showed the results of clinical studies in patients with shoulder stiffness and somatic symptoms and their symptoms were improved by adjusting the sleeping posture to be the smoothest turn over using an optimal pillow. This chapter introduces the basic researches to prove the theory underlying these clinical outcomes. The supine posture can be divided into static and dynamic ones. Static sleeping postures are the supine and lateral positions and dynamic sleeping postures are turning over.

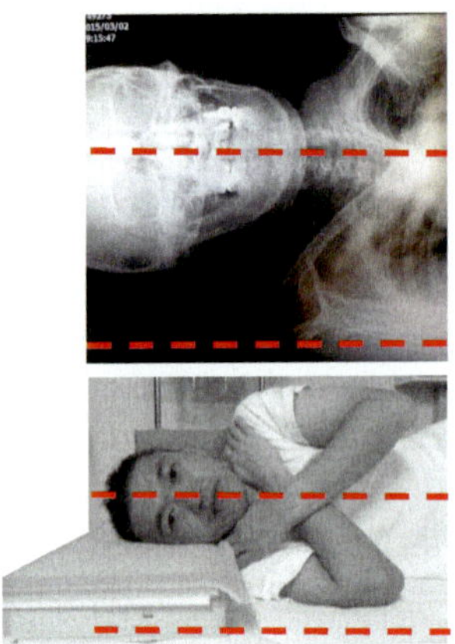

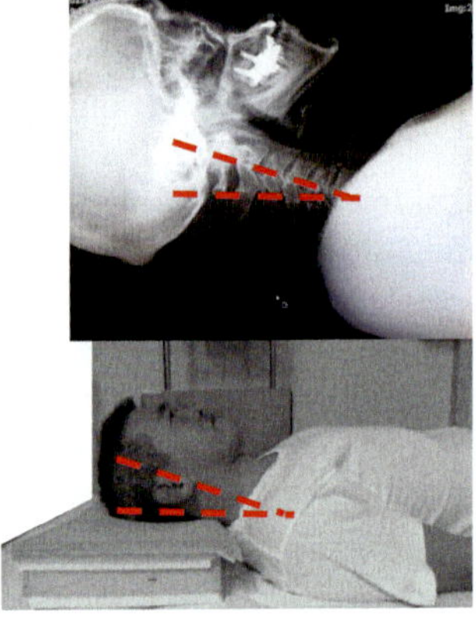

1st step: In lateral position 2nd step: In supine position

Set up for Spinal Sleep method (SSS method) is a method adjusting the height of -pillow for each person.

1st step: In the lateral position, the pillow height is adjusted so that the axis of head and trunk of the subject is aligned in parallel with the bed surface.

2nd step: In the supine position, the cervical spine is held at an angle of approximately 15 degrees anterior tilt from the bed surface.

3rd step: In the dynamic motion, we check how smoothly the subject is able to turn over according to the different height of pillow, adjusting increments and decrements of 5mm.

Finally, the pillow height that enables the subject to turn over most smoothly is the optimal adjusted pillow.

Fig. 5.1 Set up for Spinal Sleep Method (SSS Method) (JP2004209099A)

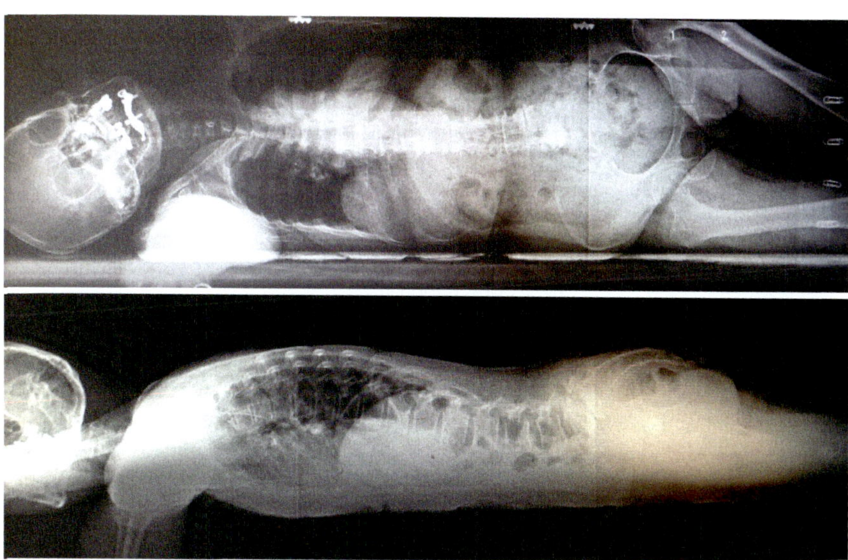

Fig. 5.2 Poor sleeping posture of total spine by X-rays. Upper: lateral position. Lower: prone position

In general, they say that a good standing posture is also ideal for the sleeping posture. However, no medical evidence supports this as far as we know. Since now, the optimal sleeping posture is still not fully elucidated. Physicians can intuitively determine that sleeping postures in Fig. 5.2 are malposture (upper, lateral position; lower, prone position) at a glance of the spinal X-ray. The supine posture during sleep depends on the bedding conditions (pillow and mattress), because the person is unconscious. The figures in Fig. 5.3 show the supine posture by the different firmness of pillows and mattresses.

Theoretically, it is optimal that side flexion angle is 0° of the coronal plane alignment or lateral position as well as coronal plane balance is 0 cm and symmetry of right and left (Fig. 5.4a). However, the optimal condition in the sagittal plane has not yet been clarified (Fig. 5.4b). 3D-CT images of different pillow heights show that the coronal plane remains symmetrical when viewed from the head with pillows of too low, optimum height, or too high (Fig. 5.5a), but the sagittal plane changes when viewed from the side (Fig. 5.5b). However, it is not possible to determine from the images which alignment is optimal for the spinal cord and nerve roots in the spinal canal (Fig. 5.5b). In order to determine the optimal supine posture, it is necessary to find a sagittal alignment, i.e., a criterion for optimal supine positioning. We analyzed the static supine posture using X-ray and MRI images and the dynamic sleeping posture using motion capture to analyze turning over movements and video observation to quantitatively evaluate actual sleep turning over.

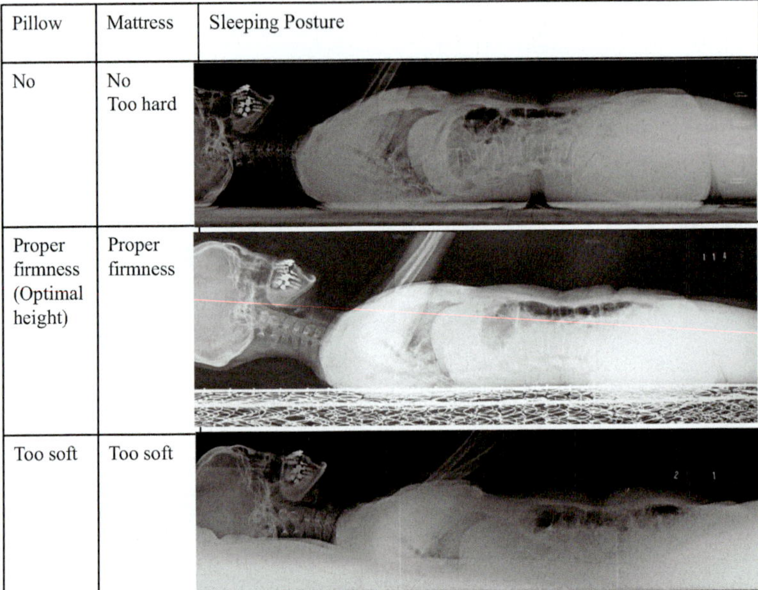

Pillow	Mattress	Sleeping Posture
No	No Too hard	
Proper firmness (Optimal height)	Proper firmness	
Too soft	Too soft	

Fig. 5.3 Sleeping postures by different firmness of pillows and mattresses

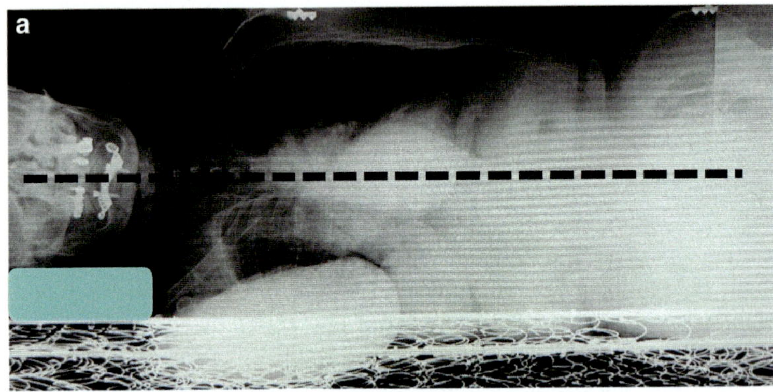

Optimal sleeping posture in the coronal plane is symmetrical

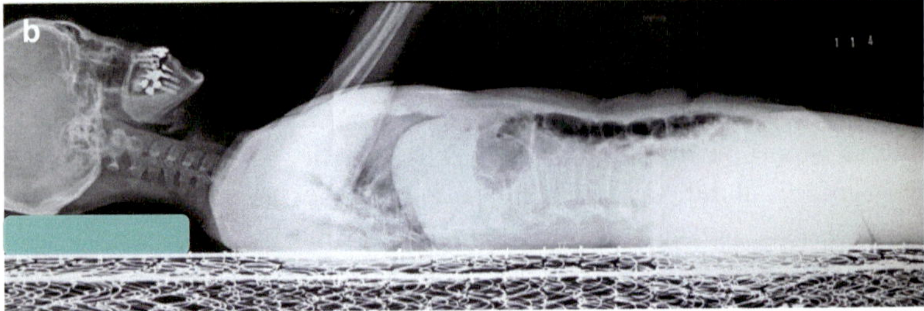

Optimal sleeping posture in sagittal plane has not been yet clarified

Fig. 5.4 Coronal and sagittal plane in sleep posture. (**a**) Coronal plane. (**b**) Sagittal plane

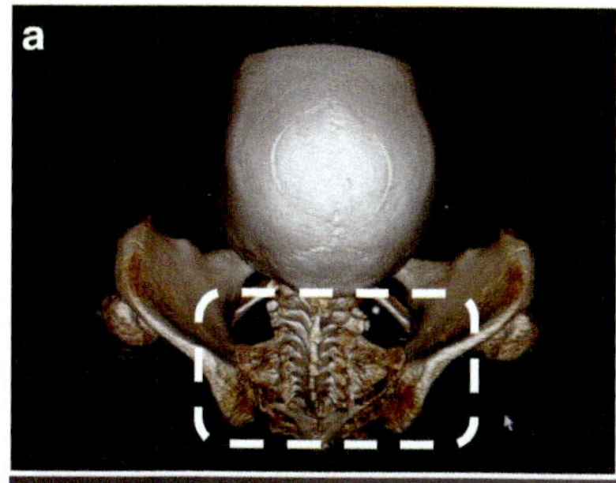

Axial view from head side
Dotted line is the outline of pillow.

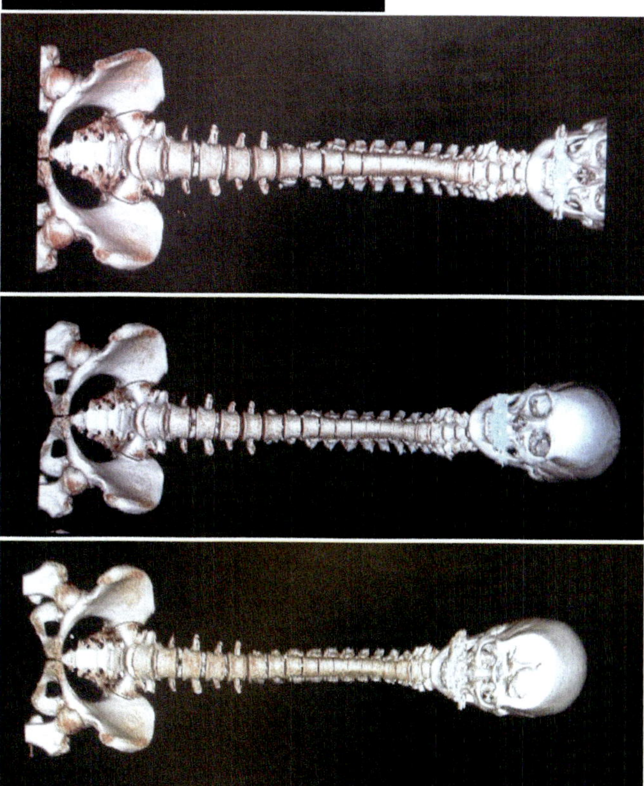

Coronal plane from above by different pillow heights
Upper, low pillow; middle, optimal height pillow; Lower, high pillow

Fig. 5.5 (**a**) 3DCT images of the total spine in coronal plane. (**b**) 3DCT images of the total spine in sagittal plane

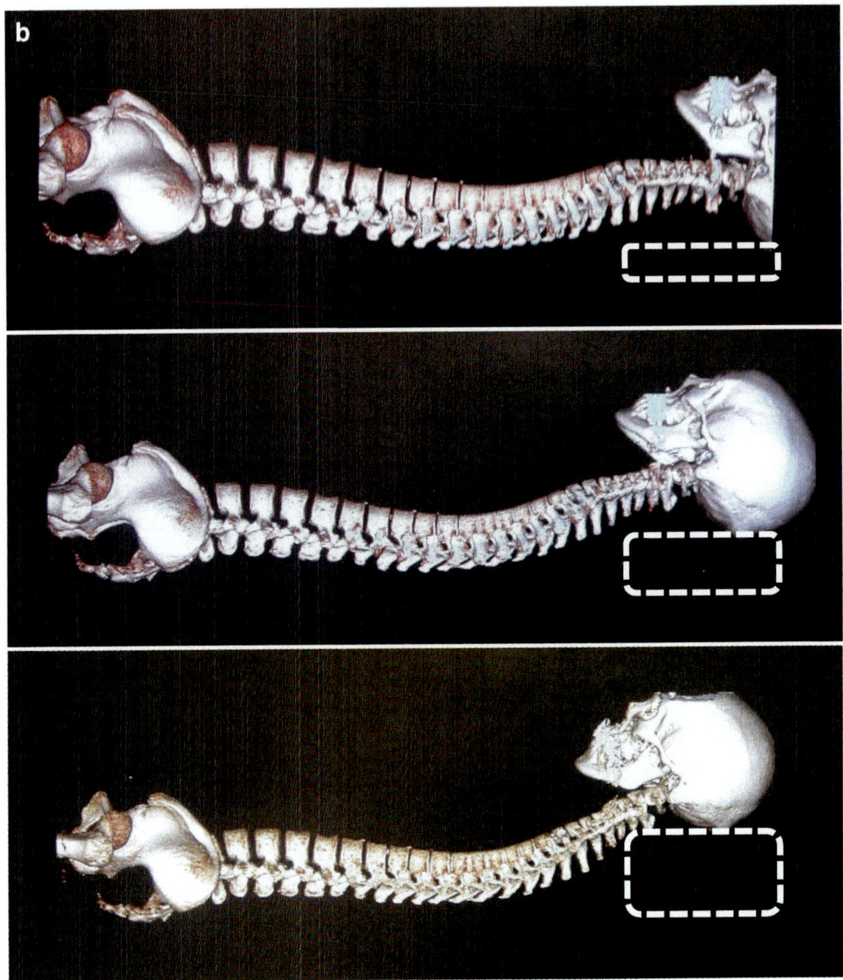

Sagittal plane from the side by different pillow heights
Upper, low pillow; middle, optimal height pillow; lower, high pillow
Dotted line is the outline of pillow.

Fig. 5.5 (continued)

5.1 Relationship Between Optimal Pillow Heights and Physiques

We performed the multiple regression analysis in 30,252 adult men and women who visited our clinic to adjust their pillows using the Set-up for Spinal Sleep (SSS) method from 2003 to 2012. The dependent variable was pillow height and independent variables were body height, body weight, and years of age (Fig. 5.6). A high multiple correlation coefficient of 0.79 was obtained, indicating that the higher the body height and the heavier the weight, the higher the pillow height. By sex, relatively little women tended to have relatively low pillows, while relatively large men tended to have high pillows. In terms of age, sometimes very high pillow heights were observed in people over 60 years of age, despite their small height and weight. They were a case of kyphosis due to rounded back, or stiffness of the spine and joints, which causes the posture to become rigid and unstretched during sleep, necessitating the use of a high pillow.

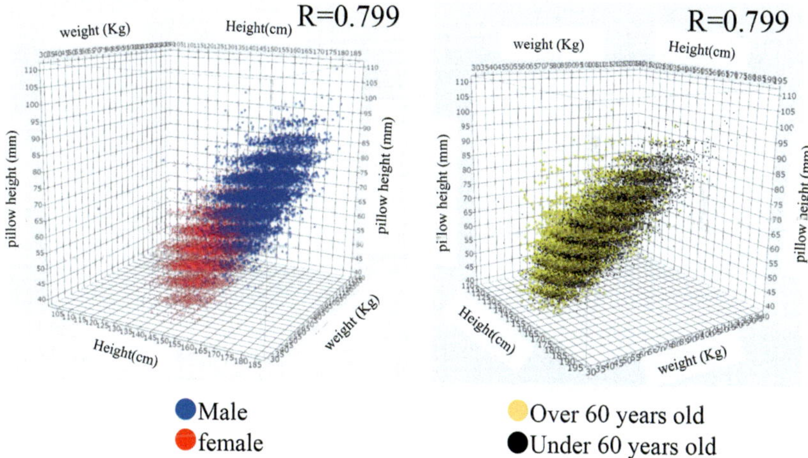

Fig. 5.6 Multiple correlation between optimal pillow height and body height/weight (by gender and age) ($N = 30{,}252$)

5.2 MRI Analysis of Cervical Spine and Cervical Spinal Cord Alignment with the Optimal Pillow: The Definition of Cervical Tilt Angle in the Supine Position

The sagittal alignment of the cervical spine and cervical cord when using the optimal pillow was analyzed using MRI. The cervical tilt angle in the supine position is an angle devised in our clinic as an index of the sagittal alignment of the cervical spine in the supine position. It is the angle between the line connecting the midpoint of the anterior margin of the foramen magnum and the posterior surface of the vertebral body of the seventh cervical vertebra and the supine plane (Fig. 5.7). It can be evaluated as an alignment from the medulla oblongata to the cervical spinal cord not only in normal persons but also in patients with subluxation of the annular axis vertebrae in rheumatoid arthritis.

We observed cervical spine alignment when using optimal pillows in 410 MRI images by gender, age, and disease in 410 patients with cervical spine disease who visited our clinic from 2004 to 2013, aged 14–93 years with a mean age of 50.5. The cervical tilt angle in the supine position was 18.1° in grand mean, and 18.1°

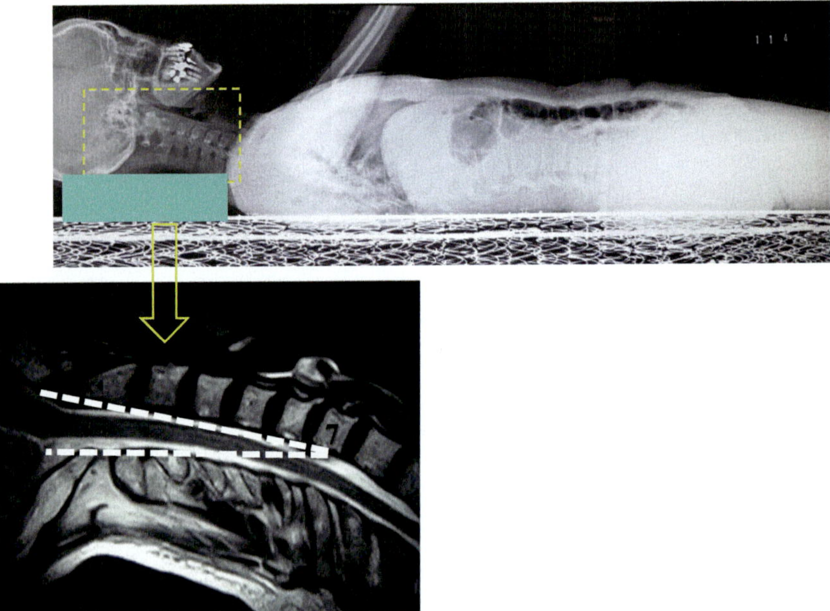

Fig. 5.7 Cervical tilt angle in the supine position by X-rays and MRI

each in males and females, with no difference by gender. By age, the distribution has single peak at 40s and ranged 17.1° to 18.9°, but not statistically significant. In comparison among groups of cervical disc degeneration, cervical disc herniation, and cervical spinal canal stenosis by MRI findings, the angles ranged 17.9° to 19.2°, but not statistically significant (Fig. 5.8). These results suggest that the cervical tilt angle in the supine position is a universal constant angle regardless of gender, age, or disease. Adjustment of cervical spine (bone) alignment in the supine position is synonymous with adjustment of cervical spinal cord (nerve) alignment. MRI shows narrowing and widening of the subarachnoid space by pillow (Fig. 5.9). To examine the anatomy of these results, we measured the anterior–posterior diameter of the subarachnoid space at the lesion. The number of cases (cases) in each lesion site were 44 for C2/3, 210 for C3/4, 309 for C4/5, 375 for C5/6, and 342 for C6/7. The anterior–posterior diameter (mm) of the subarachnoid space with no pillow/optimal pillow at each height was 8.98/9.16 for C2/3, 9.19/9.41 for C3/4, 9.17/9.55 for C4/5, 8.84/9.34 for C5/6 and 9.19/9.54 for C6/7. Subarachnoid space increased with the use of the optimal pillow at all disc levels ($P < 0.01$). The differences were 0.18 for C2/3, 0.22 for C3/4, 0.39 for C4/5, 0.50 for C5/6, and 0.45 for C6/7, with a greater increase for C5/6 and 6/7, the lower cervical spine. Both male and female patients showed a significant increase with the optimal pillow. By age, all showed significant differences except C3/4 in the 20s, C3/4 in the 30s, and C2/3 in the 70s. By MRI findings, cervical disc degeneration, cervical disc herniation, and cervical spinal canal stenosis all increased more in the lower cervical spine lesion area. Characteristically, the largest increases of 0.54 and 0.41 were observed in C5/6, the most common stenosis area in cervical disc herniation and cervical spinal canal stenosis, respectively (Fig. 5.10). The

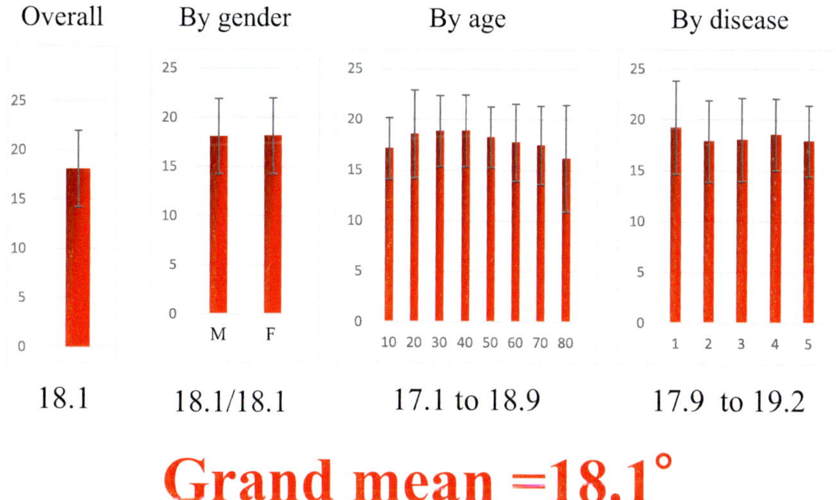

Fig. 5.8 Mean cervical tilt angle in the supine position (MRI) Overall, by sex, age, and disease (mean ± SD) ($N = 410$)

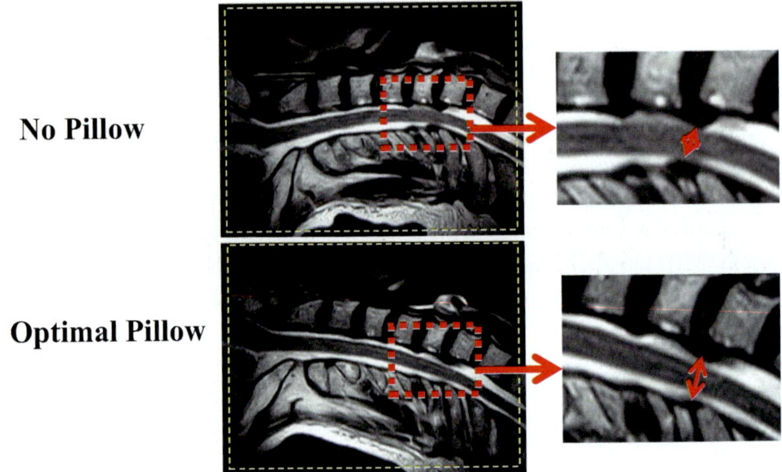

Upper row: No pillow, stenosis of the subarachnoid space
Lower row: with optimal pillow, dilatation of the subarachnoid space

Fig. 5.9 Stenosis and dilatation of the subarachnoid space caused by different pillow heights

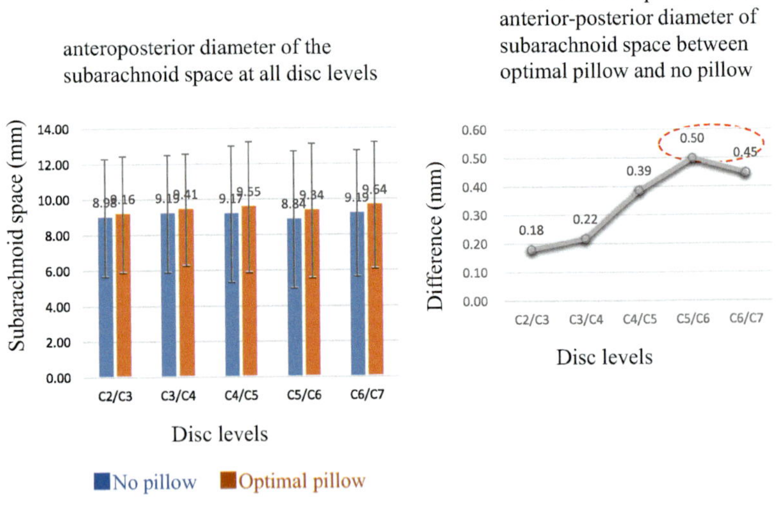

Significantly increased anteroposterior diameter of the subarachnoid space at all disc levels.
The difference between optimal pillow and no pillow was greatest at C5/6 and 6/7.

Fig. 5.10 Dilatation of the anterior–posterior diameter of the subarachnoid space with optimal pillow ($N = 410$)

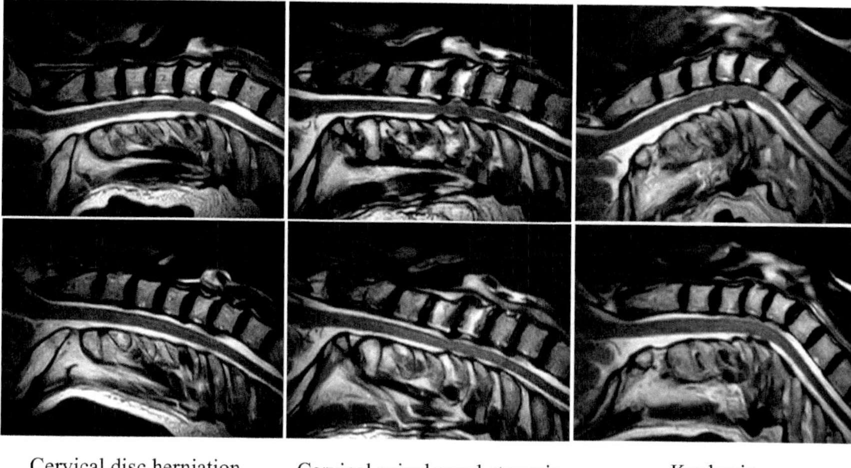

Fig. 5.11 Disease-specific comparison of MRI images. Upper: No pillow. Lower: Optimal pillow

comparison of spinal alignment and subarachnoid space of the three diseases (cervical disc herniation, cervical spinal canal stenosis, and kyphosis) in no pillow and optimal pillow by MRI images is shown in Fig. 5.11. The optimal pillow reduced the compression of the cervical spinal cord at the lesion in the static supine position, suggesting that nerve rest was maintained.

5.3 X-Ray Analysis of Sagittal Spino-Pelvic Alignment (SSPA) with the Optimal Pillow

Sagittal alignment of the cervicothoracolumbar spine and pelvis in the supine posture was analyzed using X-ray. Since no evaluation method for Sagittal Spine-Pelvic Alignment (SSPA) in the supine position is available, five parameters used in the standing posture evaluation: Sagittal Balance (SB), Ishihara Index (Cervical Kyphosis Index) (II), Thoracic Kyphosis Angle (TK), Lumbar Kyphosis Angle (LL), and Pelvic Tilt (PT) (Fig. 5.12). The patients were observed in the supine position at the optimal pillow height for the smoothest turn over in bed. Although the C7 Plumb Line (C7PL) is used to evaluate SB in the standing position, no corresponding reference line in the supine position is available. The C7HL is a straight line drawn from the posterior surface of the C7 vertebral body to a line parallel to the supine surface. The C7PL is extended cephalad and is also used as a reference for the evaluation of cervical alignment in the supine position (Fig. 5.13).

The mean (±SD, *P* value) of SPA in standing and supine positions is compared (Fig. 5.14). SB is the distance from the C7 Plumb Line (C7PL) to the Hip Axis Vertical Line (HAVL). The case that C7PL is located in front of HA is indicated by (+) and the case that C7PL is located behind HA is indicated by (−). C7PL. The

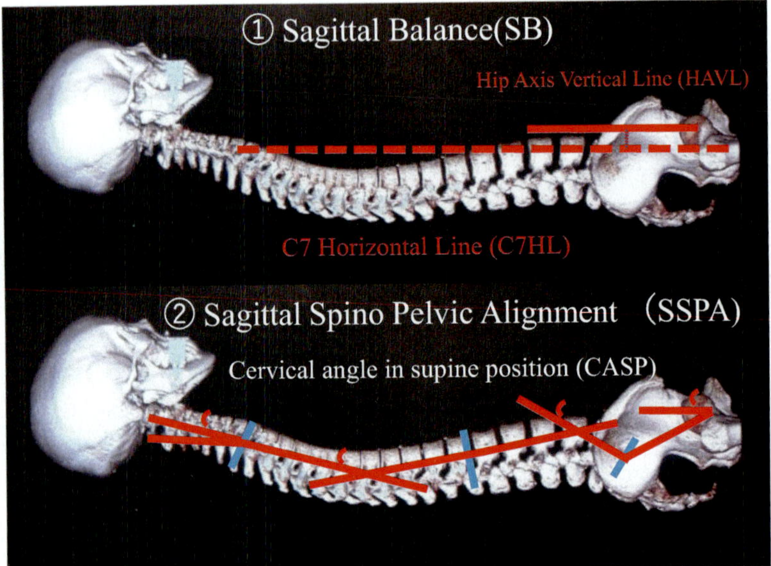

Fig. 5.12 Five parameters in the standing position assessment were used to evaluate sleep posture

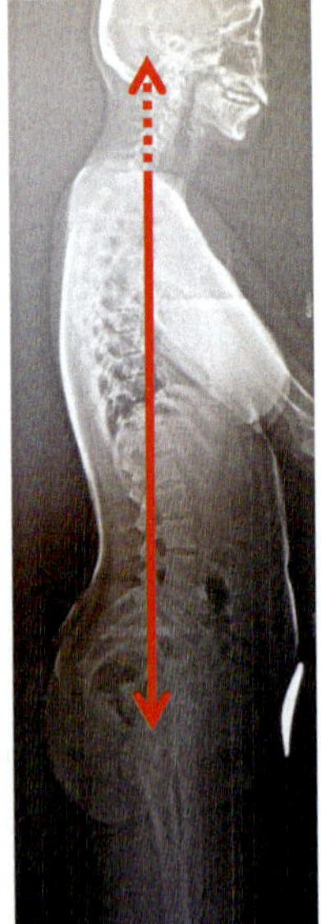

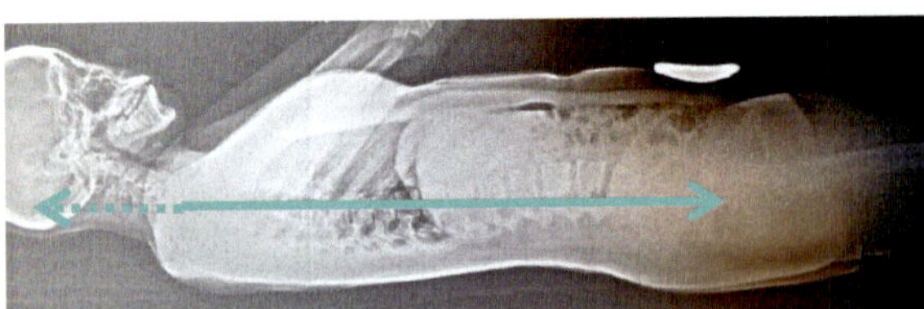

Fig. 5.13 C7 plumb line (C7PL) and C7 horizontal line (C7HL)

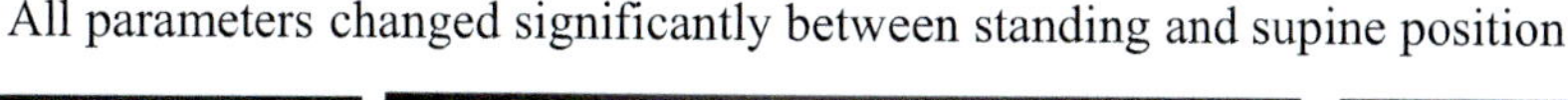

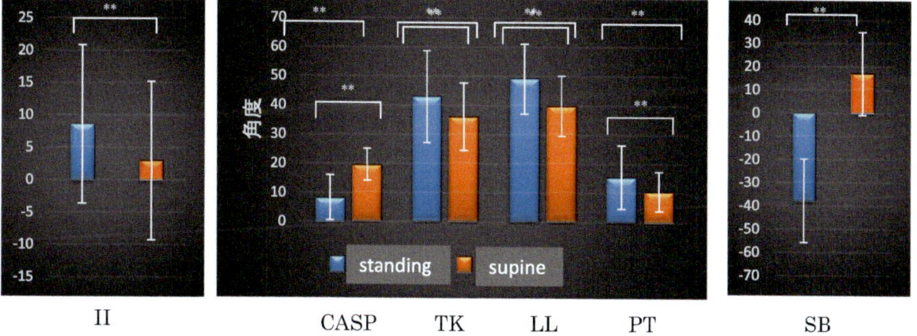

II CASP TK LL PT SB

Ishihara Index(II) , Cervical tilt angle in supine position(CASP), Thoracic kyphosis(TK) ,Lumbar lordosis(LL) , Pelvic Tilt (PT), Sagittal Balance(SB)

Fig. 5.14 Comparison of standing and supine position parameters ($N = 51$)

reference line for the supine position was defined as a straight line drawn parallel to the supine surface from C7. A total of 51 subjects, 15 males and 36 females, ages between 4 and 89 years (mean 49.1 years), were evaluated. The mean changes in standing and supine positions are: on SB, −37.85 ± 38.87 mm, 16.99 ± 17.85 mm ($P < 0.01$); on II +8.62° ± 18.12°, +2.95° ± 12.21° ($P < 0.01$); on TK +42.86° ± 15.81°, +35.96° ± 11.72° ($P < 0.01$);on LL +49.05° ±12.12°, +39.66° ± 10.5° ($P < 0.01$); and on PT +15.47° ± 11.00°, +10.44° ± 6.92° ($P < 0.01$). By age, SB showed a negative balance in all ages except 80 s in the standing position, but in the supine position, SB showed a 0 to positive balance in all ages. II was lower in the supine position than in the standing position for all ages. In the supine position, II was around 0 in 0s to 60s, but suddenly became higher in 70s and 80s. The TK was lower in the lying position than in the standing position for all ages except for those in 40s. The LL was higher in the lying position than in the standing position for all ages. The PT was lower in the supine position than in the standing position for all ages.

The results indicated that the curvature in the supine position decreased and approached a straight line compared with that in the standing position. The sagittal curvature of the normal spine in the standing position provides flexibility in locomotion and axial load-bearing capacity, i.e., rigidity and stability to maintain the standing position. Conversely, in the supine position, no axial load applied to the spine, and motion is in the rotational direction of turn over. Therefore, the tendency toward straightening of the spine due to a decrease in II, TK, and LL is considered an ideal change that decreases the eccentricity of the center of rotation for turning and facilitates turn over. In the 70s and 80s, when disc degeneration, spinal deformity, or compression fracture causes kyphosis or joint contracture, SSPA in the supine positions are different compared to those without deformity, such as high SB, high II, high TK, and high PT. We believe that the supine position, or SSPA, should be adjusted to enable smooth turn over, taking age and individual deformity into consideration. The comparison of SSPA in the standing and supine positions according to age is shown in the X-ray image (Fig. 5.15a, b). In the standing position, SB increases with age, resulting in a poor posture. In the supine position, SB increases as well, but is smaller than in the standing position.

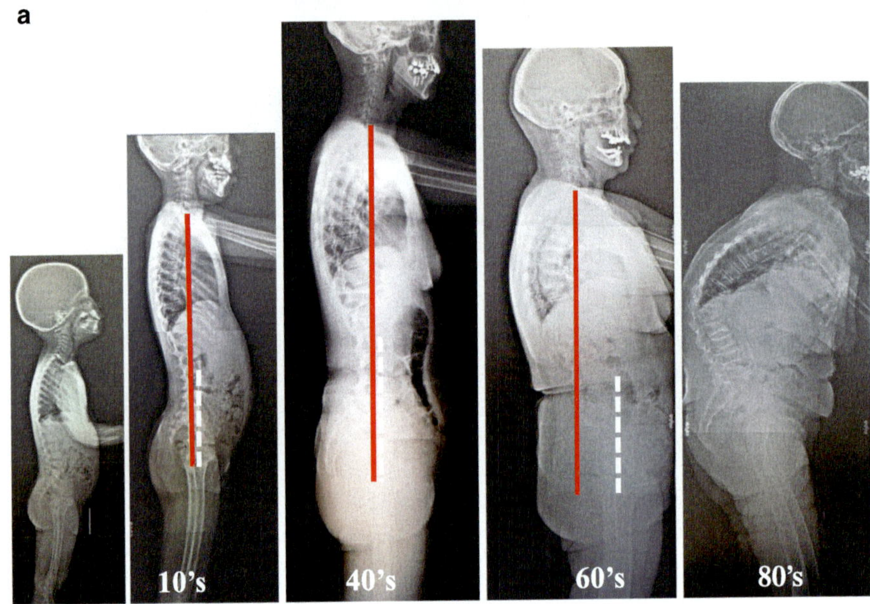

Fig. 5.15 (**a**) Age-specific SSPA in the standing position. (**b**) Age-specific SSPA in sleeping posture

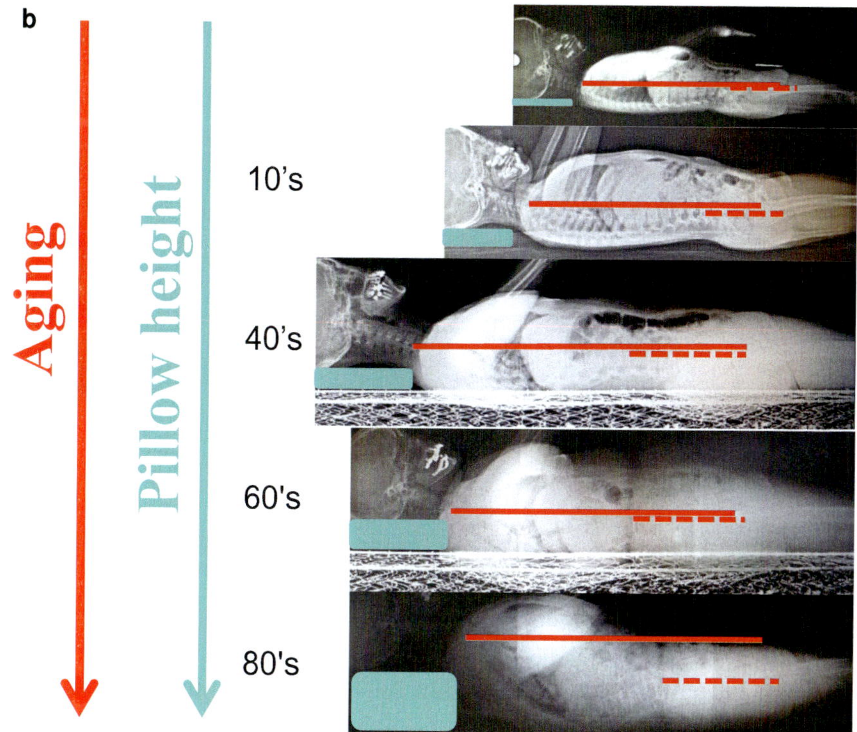

In the supine position, sagittal balance (SB) distance increases with age, but SB is less than the standing positon
Solid line C7HL Dotted line：HAVL

Fig. 5.15 (continued)

5.4 Four-Dimensional Motion Analysis of Turning Over with the Optimal Pillow

In order to quantitatively evaluate the smoothness of the turning over motion, we performed a 4D motion analysis of the turning motion using the motion capture system Vicon 8 to visualize the virtual body axes, while it had been evaluated macroscopically (Fig. 5.16). The experiment was conducted at the Creative Laboratory, Tokyo University of Technology. A total of 16 subjects were healthy volunteers of the university. Three conditions were used for the pillow: optimal pillow, no pillow, and high pillow. Two conditions were used for the bed: a good condition (mattress with moderate firmness) and a bad condition (too soft mattress). Thirty-seven optical markers were attached to the head, shoulders, pelvis, and lower limbs. Eighteen

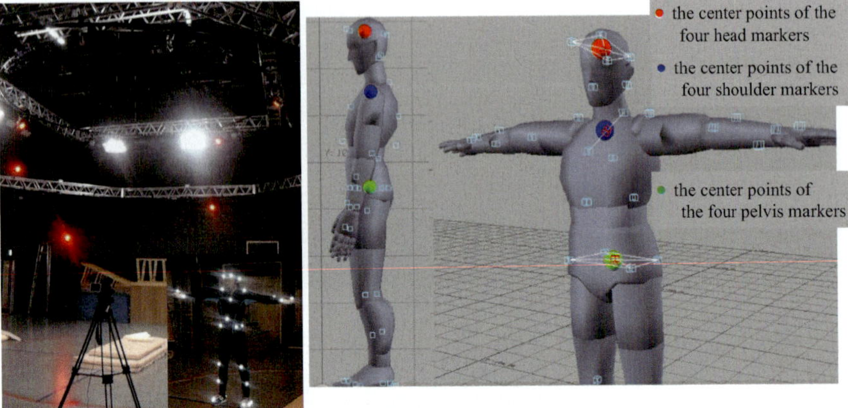

The Vicon 8 motion capture system

Three points of the head, chest and lumbar region creating a virtual body axis

Fig. 5.16 Four-dimension motion analysis using a motion capture system

optical infrared cameras were used to film the turning over movements and acquire the trajectory data of the markers. The motion picture in Fig. 5.17a, Video 5.1 was edited from the 4D coordinate data, and the smoothness of turning over was evaluated qualitatively.

The smoothness of turning over in sleep by pillow heights and mattress firmness can be qualitatively evaluated. When an optimal pillow and a mattress of good firmness were used, turning over was smooth. With a low pillow or a high pillow, the turning over was not smooth regardless of firmness of mattress. Computer analysis of the turning over motion was performed to obtain the velocity and acceleration. The frequency spectrum was analyzed using the Fast Fourier Transform (FFT) to separate the low-frequency components representing the smoothness and the high-frequency components representing the non-smoothness and quantified them. An example of a quantitative comparison of the smoothness of turning over in sleep according to pillow suitability is shown in (Fig. 5.17b). In the velocity graph, the circled waveform is relatively smooth during turning over in the good condition, but not in the bad condition. In all cases, when the low-frequency components were determined by the frequency spectrum, it changed significantly ($P < 0.01$) in the means of 0.193 (19.3%) for the good condition and 0.168 (16.8%) for the bad condition, allowing for a quantitative comparison of turning over (Fig. 5.17c).

Next, the virtual body axis, which is the center of rotation of turning over, was visualized from the 4-dimensional coordinate data (Fig. 5.18, Video 5.2). The virtual body axis was defined as a line passing through the center points of each of the four markers of the head, shoulders, and pelvis. The line connecting the centers of the head and the shoulder is called the head–neck virtual body axis, and the line

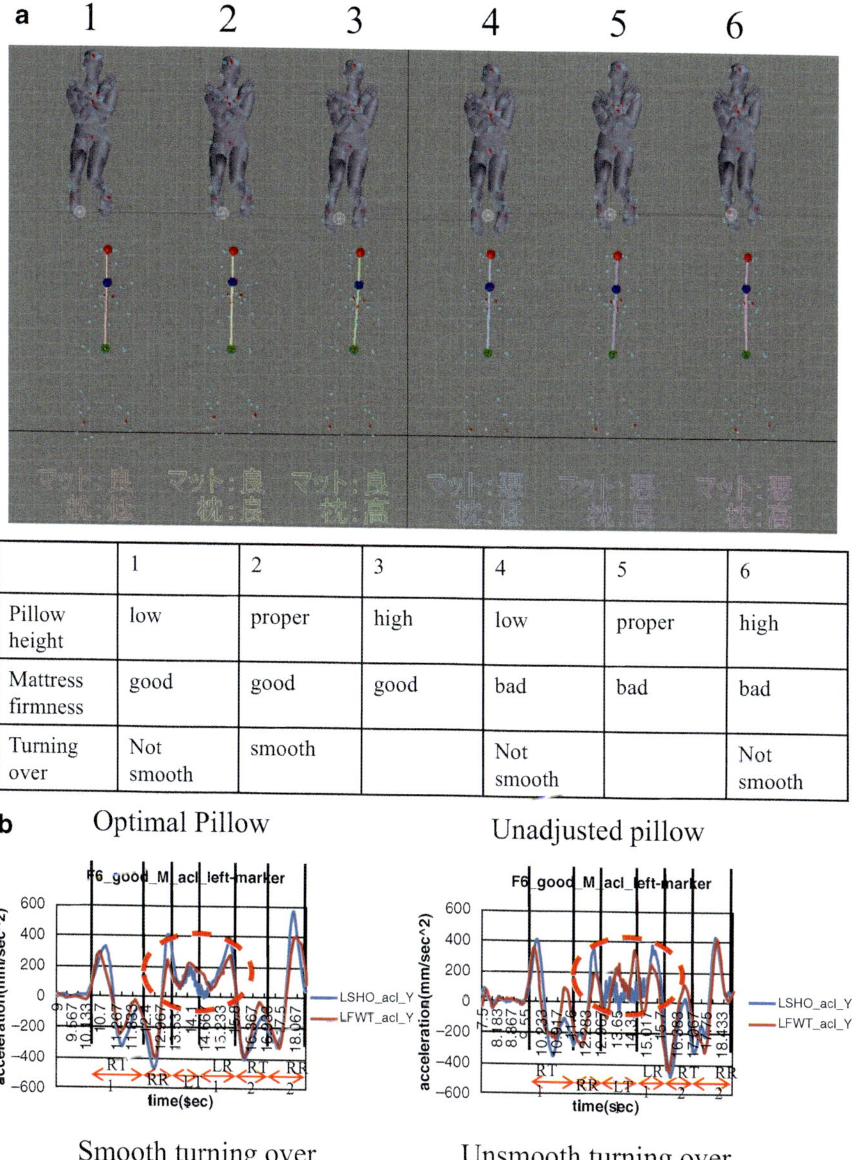

	1	2	3	4	5	6
Pillow height	low	proper	high	low	proper	high
Mattress firmness	good	good	good	bad	bad	bad
Turning over	Not smooth	smooth		Not smooth		Not smooth

Fig. 5.17 (**a**) Qualitative evaluation of the smoothness of turning over by different pillow heights and mattress firmness. (**b**) Quantitative analysis 1: acceleration analysis analyzing smoothness of turning over by pillow adaptation. (**c**) Quantitative analysis 2: frequency spectrum analysis analyzing smoothness of turning by pillow adaptation

c

Optimum Pillow

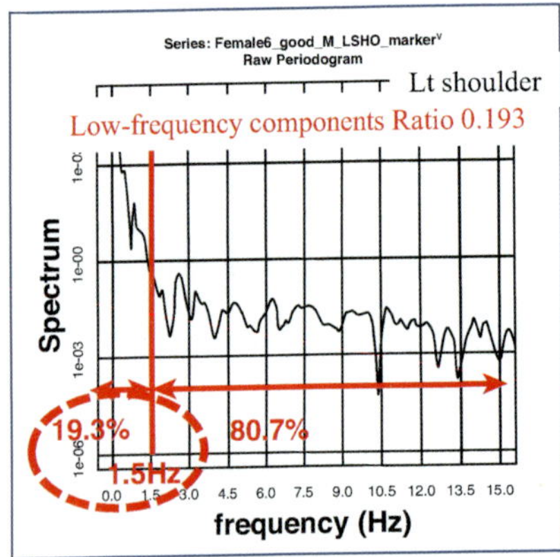

Smooth turning over

Unadjusted pillow

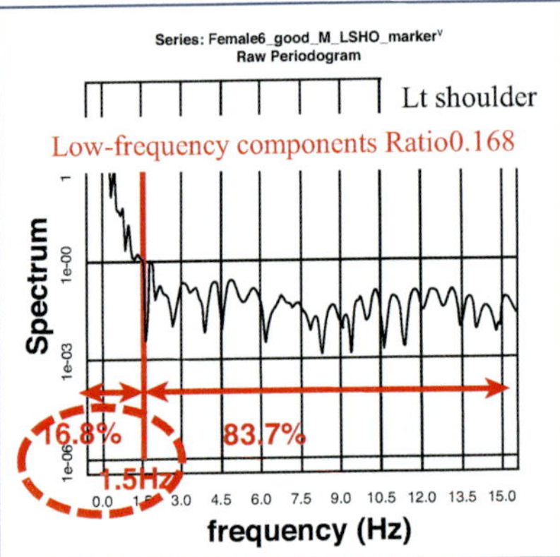

Unsmooth turning over

Fig. 5.17 (continued)

Real image

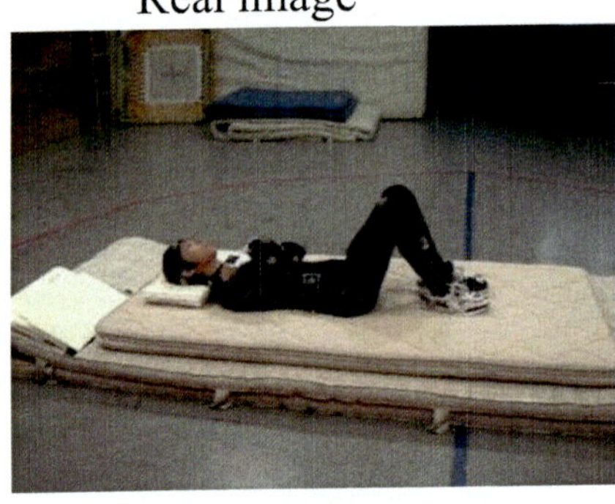

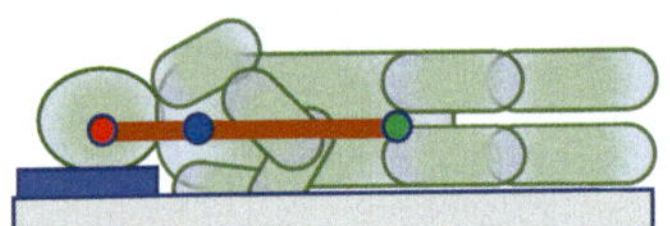

Computer graphic image

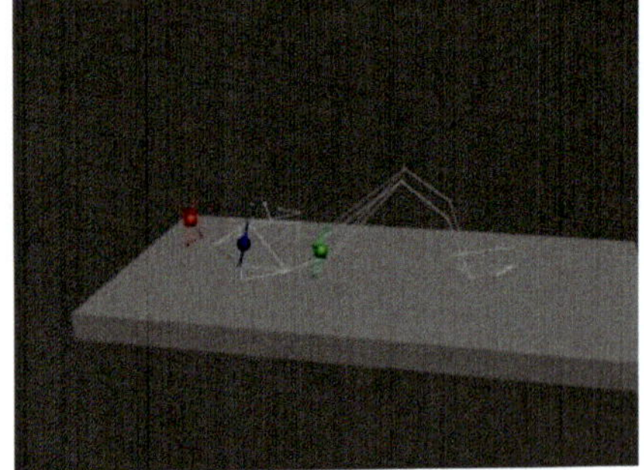

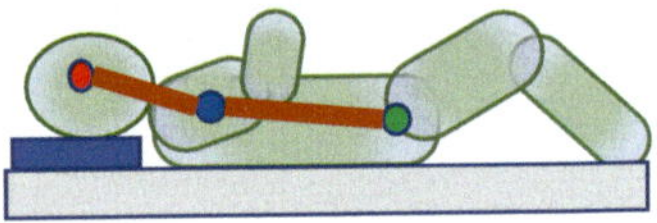

Fig. 5.18 Visualization of virtual body axes from 4D coordinate data

connecting the centers point of the shoulder and the pelvis is called the thoracolumbar pelvis virtual body axis. The angle between the line extending the thoracolumbar-pelvic virtual body axis linearly toward the head and the head and neck virtual body axis was defined as the head and neck body axis angle. The mean head–neck body axis angle in smooth turning determined quantitatively by frequency spectrum analysis in 16 subjects was 18.1° ± 3.71°, which approximated the supine cervical tilt angle of 16.8° ± 5.36° in the X-ray analysis ($P = 0.15$).

Additionally, the thoracolumbar-pelvic virtual body axis was compared with the C7 plumb line (C7PL), which is the reference line in the supine position for X-ray analysis. The distance of the perpendicular line from the starting point of the thoracolumbar-pelvic virtual body axis to the C7PL (body axis-PL distance) and the angle between the virtual body axis and the C7PL (body axis-PL angle) were measured. The body axis-PL distance ranged from 0 to 3.0 mm, and the body axis-PL angle was $-1.58° \pm 5.54°$. The virtual body axis and C7PL were nearly coincident or parallel. In smooth turning over, as a result, the thoracolumbar-pelvic virtual body axis was shown to be parallel to the supine plane.

These results suggest that the head and neck and thoracolumbar pelvis virtual body axes, which are the rotation centers of turning over in motion capture analysis, may approximate the sagittal plane alignment of the cervicothoracolumbar pelvis in the human body in X-ray analysis.

5.5 Video Analysis of Turning Over During Sleeping

Since the analysis of turning over movements using the motion capture is a simulation-based study in the awake state, in this study, we observed and quantitatively evaluated the features of actual turning over movements in the video analysis of the sleeping state during sleep.

The subjects were 17 healthy volunteers, mean age 42.5 years, 9 males and 8 females. The subjects were video taped for 3 days using a custom-made mattress named MAKURAinBED® (MinB) (JP201619726A) (Fig. 5.19, Video 5.3) with individually adjusted pillow height and bed sinkage using the Set-up for Spinal Sleep-Total (SSS-T) method (Fig. 5.20). The recorded videos were visually analyzed to determine the supine posture based on the angles of three turning patterns (head, body, and head-body simultaneous), and the average number of turning over (T) and the mean interval of turning overs (TI) were calculated.

Result 1: The mean sleep duration was 6 h. Number of Head (H) turning over was 24 (range: 5–56), number of body (B) turning over was 16 (range: 3–47), number of Head and Body (H & B), head and body at the same time, turning over was 15 (range: 2–47) (Fig. 5.21). As a result, number of turning over in H was 9 times more frequent than that in H & B, and number of turning over in B was 1 time more frequent than that in H & B. When H & B was compared by gender, the difference between men and women was 4 (men, 17; women, 13), but not significant ($P = 0.53$) (Fig. 5.22).

Result 2: TI was 15 and 23 min for H and B, respectively. The time distribution of TI for H & B showed that the frequencies of two consecutive turn overs occurred within 10 min were 14 (60%) for H and 9 (56%) for B (Fig. 5.23). The subjects with average, high, and low number of turn overs are shown in Fig. 5.24.

Result 3: When the number of turning over was divided into sleep time periods (first and last halves of sleeping time), T in H was 13 in the first half and 11 in the last half, and no significant difference was observed between the first and last halves. T in B was 8 in the first half and 7 in the last half, and no significant difference was

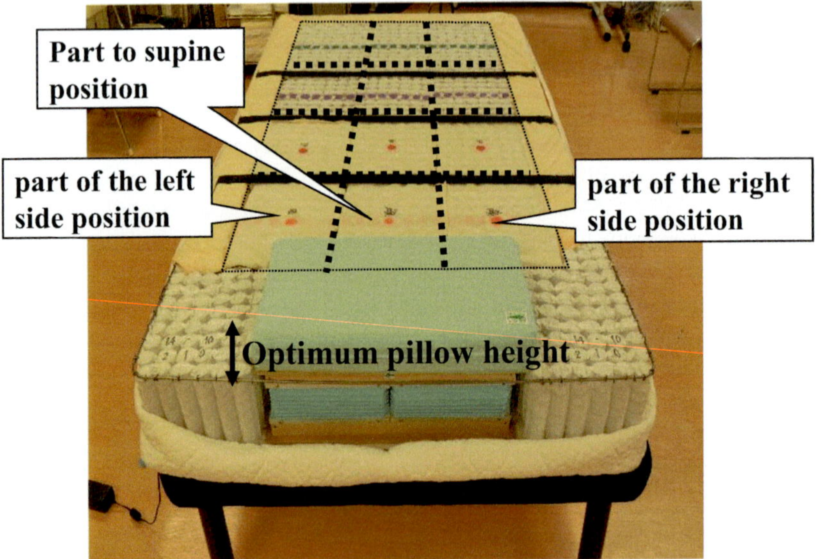

1. device MAKURAinBED ® to implement the SSS-T method
- The pillow elevator can adjust the pillow height in 1 mm intervals.
- 3 rows x 4 columns = 12 coil spring units with different spring constants, each point of which can be adjusted individually.
- Localisation for supine and lateral positions.

2. Adjustment procedure
- First, in the supine position, adjust the middle row coil unit to the four points (points are C7, Th7, L4 and S).
- Next, in the side lying position, adjust the left and right side coil units at two points (acromion and greater trochanter).
- Finally, the smoothness of turning over is checked.

Fig. 5.19 MAKURAinBED ® (MinB) (JP201619726A)

also observed between them. Five (29%) of the subjects turned more in the first half, 11 (65%) in the last half, and 1 (6%) was the same in both halves (Fig. 5.25).

Many preceding sleep observational studies have not specified the details of bedding conditions, and it cannot be denied the possibility that the bedding used (pillow and mattress) had somewhat affected the results of studies. Therefore, we determined the bedding conditions that facilitated individual turning over by using the SSS method (Fig. 5.1) to maintain a certain optimal sleep posture and then conducted observations.

Step 1. static posture adjustment
in the supine and lateral position

1) Supine position: sagittal view
- Supine cervical tilt angle approximately15°
- Subjective and objective adjustment of thoracic kyphosis, lumbar kyphosis and sacral alignment
- Adjustment points are C7, Th7, L4 and S

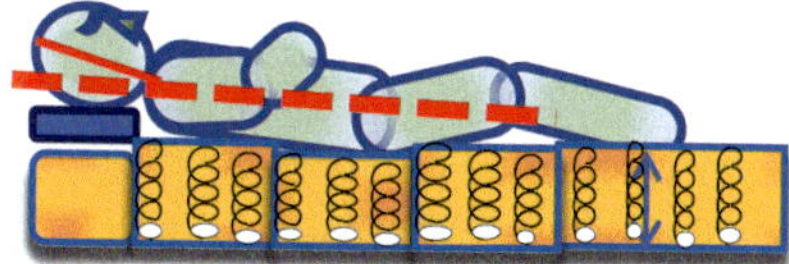

2) Lateral position: coronal view
- The axis of the head to trunk is aligned in parallel with the bed surface

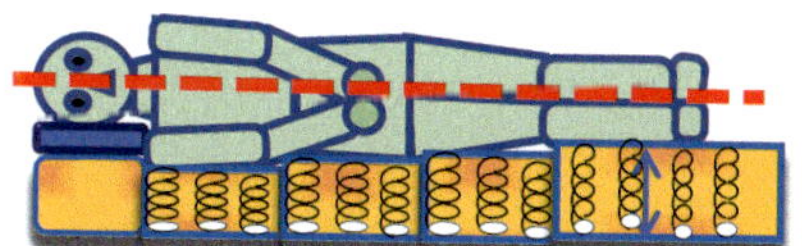

Step 2: Dynamic posture adjustment
In the turning over

merkmals to check smoothness of turning over are acromion and greater trochanter

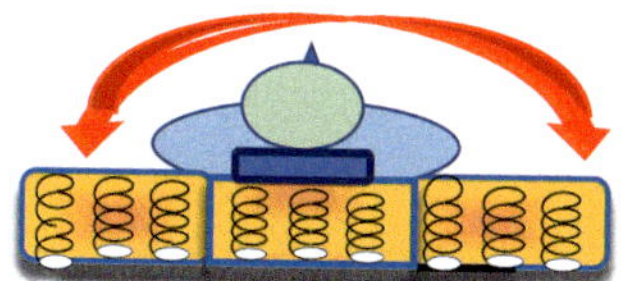

Fig. 5.20 Method of Set-up for Spinal Sleep-Total (SSS-T)

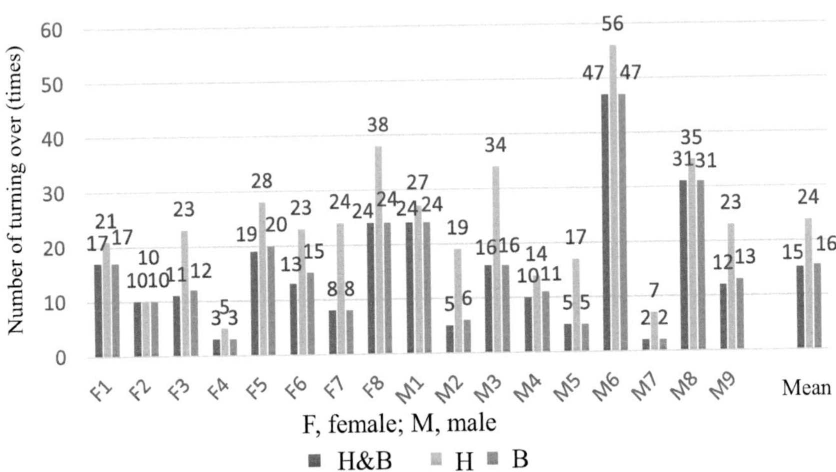

Fig. 5.21 Number of turnover head and body ($N = 17$)

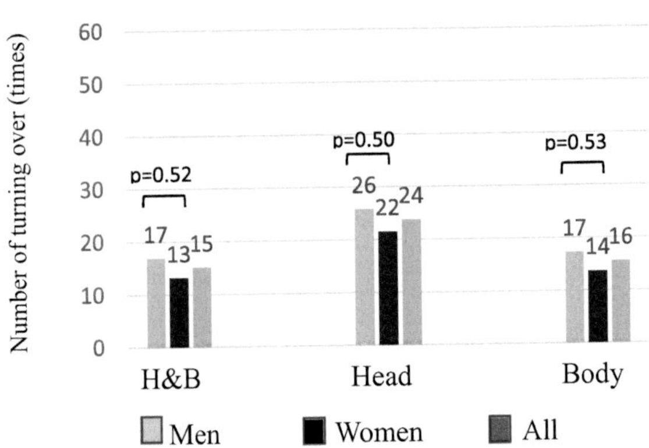

Fig. 5.22 Comparison of the number of turn over in men and women ($N = 17$)

Generally, it is said T becomes around 20 in the sleep medicine and our results consisted with it. However, in the study, we revealed the differences among H, B, and H & B, and individuals as well. The TI was within 10 min for about 60% of the subjects, and subjects who turned over frequently indicated a large difference between within 10 min and over.

There are two types of sleep: REM sleep and non-REM sleep. The transition from non-REM to REM sleep is sometimes triggered by body movements (turning

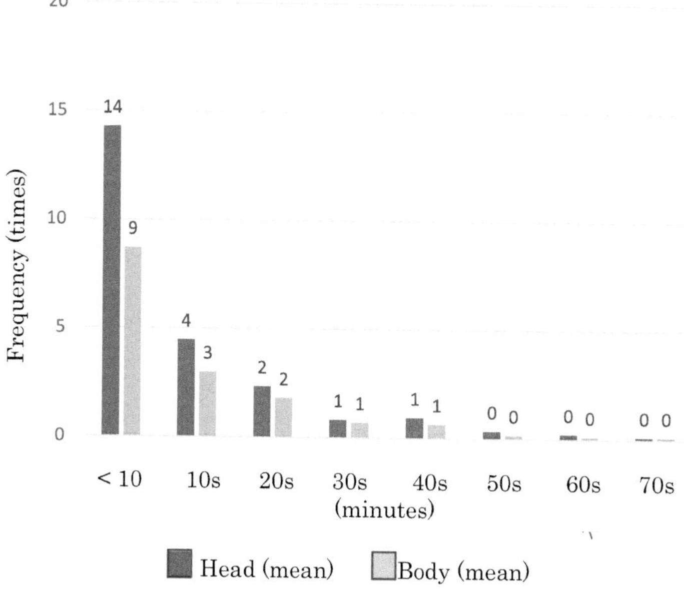

Mean sleeping duration: 6 hours
Mean interval: 15 min. for head and 23 min. for body

Fig. 5.23 Distribution of Interval time of turn over ($N = 17$)

over), and turning over may be engaged on these two sleeps. It is said that number of turning over tends to increase at dawn because non-REM sleep decreases and REM sleep increases and arouses. Results of our study also showed a tendency for more people to turn over in the last half of their sleep, compared to the first.

Although studies on "turning over in sleep" have been reported in the two fields of the rehabilitation medicine and the sleep medicine, their methods perceiving and analyzing this phenomenon are quite difference. In the rehabilitation medicine, turning over is considered a kind of "changing position" or "rotating movement" during wakefulness, and therefore motion analysis is conducted. Converesly, in the sleep medicine, turning over is considered as "body movement" during sleep, especially coarse movements of the trunk and extremities, and physiological analysis such as electromyography is performed. We have focused on the relationship between "rotating movement" during wakefulness in the rehabilitation medicine and "body movement" during sleep in the sleep medicine. We hypothesized that if the bedding (pillow and mattress) is adjusted for optimal rotation during wakefulness, optimal turning over can also be achieved during sleep. As a first step, we obtained basic data by observing the head and body separately in order to quantify the characteristics of turning over during sleep.

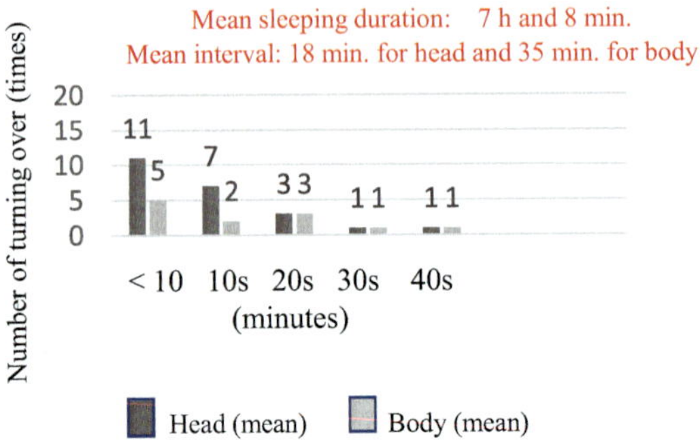

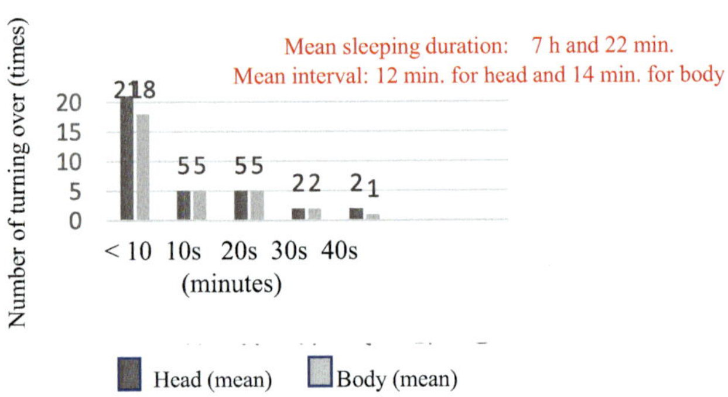

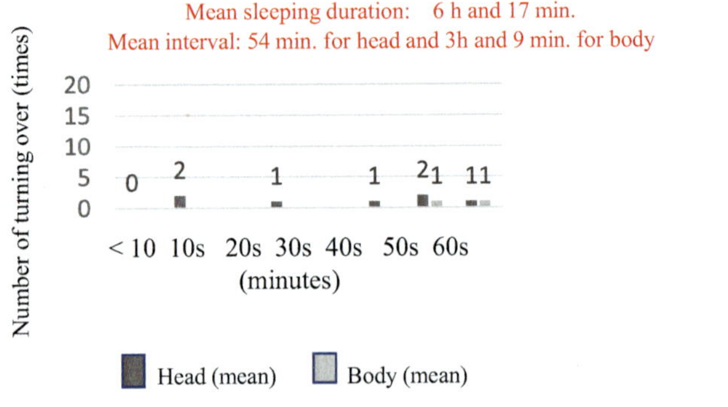

Fig. 5.24 Interval distributions by subject sub-group

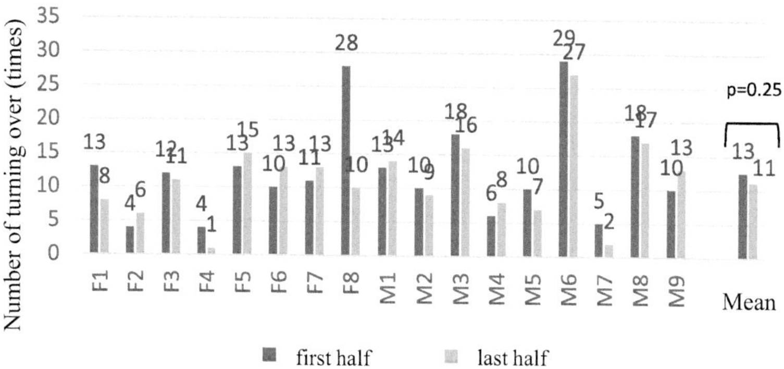

Number of head turn over by sleeping duration (first and last halves)

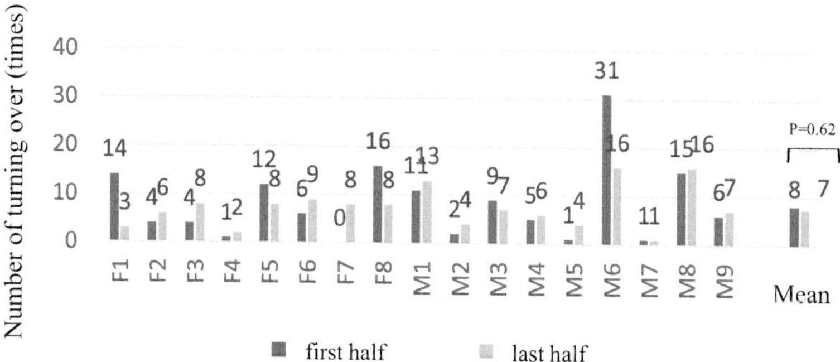

Number of body turn over by sleeping duration (first and last halves)

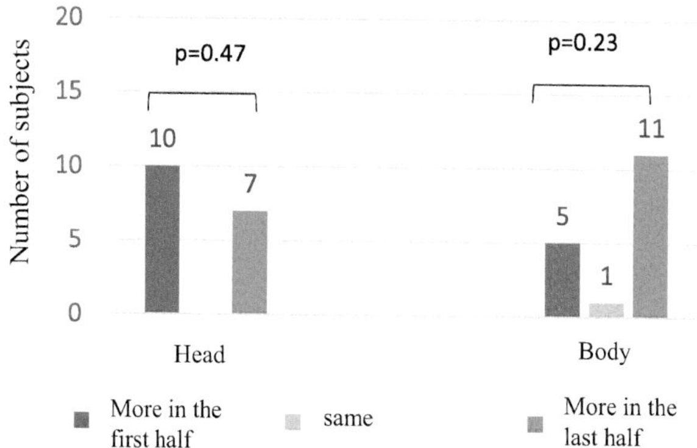

Time zone when more head and body turn over occurs (first and last halves)

Fig. 5.25 Time zone and number of turn over ($N = 17$)

5.6 All-Night Observation and Analysis of Sleep Position and Sleep Posture Control by Bedding Adjustment

5.6.1 Introduction

In recent years, mattress designs used during sleep to prevent and treat sleep-related skeletal muscular system problems have been discussed. In 2019, Duo Wai-chi Wong et al. [1] reviewed the recent trends, research methodologies, and determinants of biomechanics researches on mattress published since 2008. In conclusion, mattress designs have strived for customization, regional features, and real-time active control to adapt to the biomechanical features of different body sizes and postures. Jordi Esquirol Caussa et al. [2] designed and validated an automated prescription model for an individualized sleep system that was developed through a single-image 2D-3D analysis and body pressure distribution, to objectively determine optimal individually designed mattress-topper-pillow combination by five different mattress densities, three different toppers, and three cervical pillows.

We also believe that in order to achieve an optimal sleep posture for persons with different physiques, it is necessary to adjust the bedding to fit each individual's body parts. We have developed the SSS-T method (Fig. 5.20), which uses X-ray spinal-pelvic alignment (SPA) measurements and motion capture analysis of turning movements to determine and adjust the pillow and bedding according to static sleep posture (supine and lateral) and dynamic sleep posture (turning over). Using the MinB bed mattress (Fig. 5.19), which was developed for use in this SSS-T method, we observed and analyzed whether it was possible to control the patient to sleep in an appropriate sleep position and sleep posture throughout the night.

5.6.2 Subjects and Methods

A total of 17 adults (9 males and 8 females), mean age 42.4 years (30–67 years), were examined using the SSS-T method to adjust the SPA in the sagittal plane in the supine position and the coronal plane in the right and left lateral positions. The MinB consists of 3 rows × 3 columns = 9 coil spring units with different spring constants that can adjust each point individually. First, the center row is used to adjust each point in the supine position, and then the left and right rows are adjusted in the lateral positions. Finally, the smoothness of turning over is checked. The bedding conditions were as follows: bedding A was adjusted for optimal pillow and the MinB bedding, and bedding B was adjusted for optimal pillow and conventional bedding at home. Videos were taken throughout the night for 3 days. The combined time course of sleep position (center column C, right column R, left column L) and sleep posture (supine position s, right side lying position r, left side lying position l) is recorded from the video (Fig. 5.26). Also shown are videos of the actual turn over in sleep observed. The percentage of time that the sleep position and sleep posture coincided (C-s, R-r, L-l) is defined as the coincidence rate, and the coincidence rates

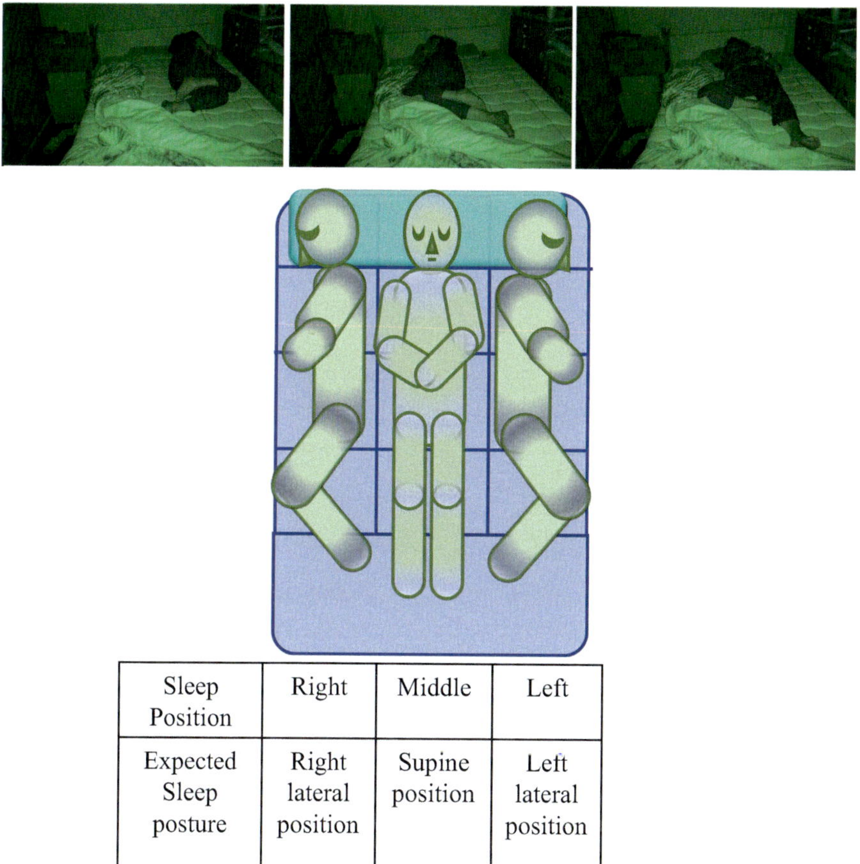

Sleep Position	Right	Middle	Left
Expected Sleep posture	Right lateral position	Supine position	Left lateral position

Bedding A: optimal pillow and the MinB bedding
Bedding B: optimal pillow and conventional bedding at home

Fig. 5.26 All-night observations of sleep position and expected sleep posture (bedding A and B), and the videos observing actual turn over in sleep. Bedding A: optimal pillow and the MinB bedding. Bedding (Video 5.4.1, Video 5.4.2, Video 5.4.3), Bedding B: optimal pillow and conventional bedding at home

(mean ± 2 SD) of A and B are compared to statistically test for significant differences (p value). The calculation of the agreement rate for the sleep position and posture sequence is shown in Fig. 5.27.

The coincidence rates in 13 (76.5%) subjects out of 17 were A > B, and in residual 4 (23.5%) subjects were B > A. The mean coincidence rates for the former 13 subjects were 0.85 ± 0.25 for A and 0.64 ± 0.38 for B. The difference between A and B was statistically significant ($P < 0.001$). The mean coincidence rates for the residual four patients were 0.28 ± 0.40 for A and 0.48 ± 0.35 for B, with no significant difference ($P > 0.05$) (Table 5.1). In the video analysis, large body movements due to prone position and breathing disorders were observed.

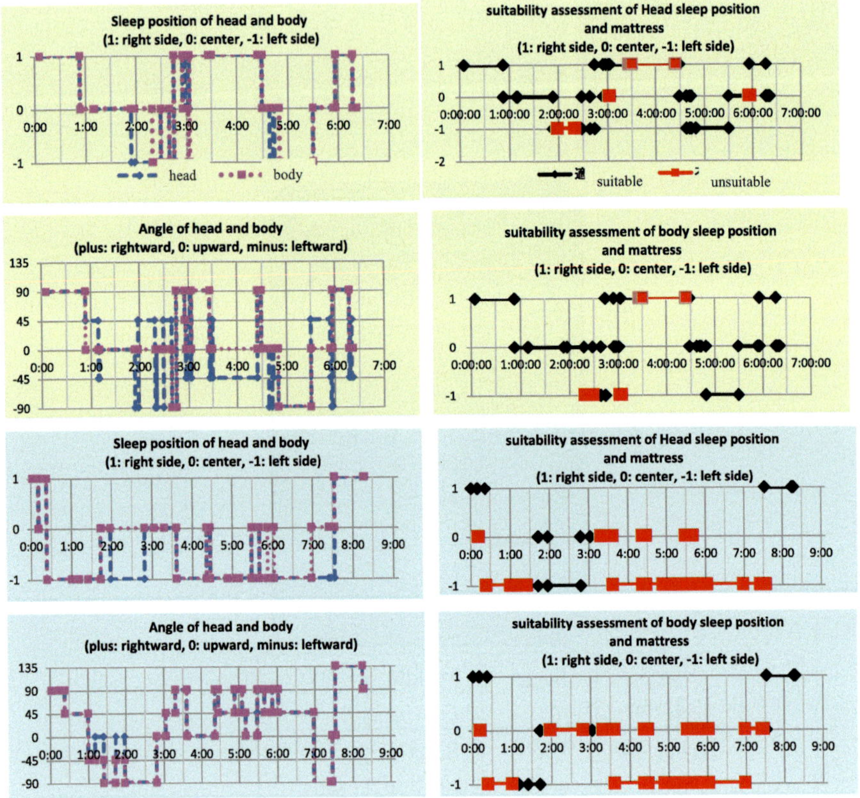

coincidence rate :
Percentage of matches between sleep position and expected sleep posture in the head and body

Case 1: Poor example
Head coincidence rate = adequate sleep time/total sleep time = 4:57/6:16 = 0.79
Body coincidence rate = adequate sleep time/total sleep time = 5:06/6:16 = 0.81

Case 2: Good example
Head coincidence rate = adequate sleep time/total sleep time = 3:13/8:16 = 0.45
Body coincidence rate = adequate sleep time/total sleep time = 2:30/8:16=0.34

Fig. 5.27 Rates of sleep position and postural coincidence ($N = 17$)

Table 5.1 Comparison of coincidence rates for mattress A and B

Coincidence rates

	Head		Body	
Subject no.	Mattress A	Mattress B	Mattress A	Mattress B
1	0.45	0.54	0.71	0.46
2	0.71	0.64	0.71	0.53
3	0.79	0.84	0.81	0.63
4	0.95	0.97	1.00	0.99
5	0.85	0.82	0.69	0.64
6	0.90	0.32	0.82	0.78
7	1.00	0.74	1.00	0.74
8	1.00	0.51	1.00	0.45
9	0.62	0.59	0.79	0.67
10	0.82	0.57	0.73	0.31
11	1.00	1.00	1.00	0.83
12	0.94	0.79	0.95	0.80
13	0.61	0.49	0.79	0.45
Mean	**0.82**	**0.67**	**0.85**	**0.64**
2SD	0.35	0.42	0.25	0.38
Result	*P*=0.021 between A and B		*P*=0.0004 between A and B	

Coincidence rates

	Head		Body	
Subject no.	Mattress A	Mattress B	Mattress A	Mattress B
14	0.45	0.67	0.34	0.58
15	0.26	0.58	0.21	0.60
16	0.59	0.76	0.53	0.53
17	0.06	0.06	0.06	0.22
Mean	**0.34**	**0.52**	**0.29**	**0.48**
2SD	0.47	0.63	0.39	0.17
Result	N.S. between mattresses A and B *p*=0.069		N.S. between mattresses A and B *p*=0.091	

5.6.3 Results

In 76.5% ($n = 13$) of subjects, the coincidence rates for bedding A were higher than that for bedding B, suggesting that all-night sleep in MinB with bedding adjustment based on our SSS-T method significantly controls sleep positions and postures.

In 23.5% ($n = 4$) of the subjects, the coincidence rates were low for both bedding A and B, with no significant difference between A and B. The result suggested that any other factors other than bedding conditions or pre-existing medical conditions had influenced. Clarification of these factors is necessary for sleep posture control in persons with problems other than bedding conditions.

In the future, we would like to increase the number of subjects to improve the reliability of the data and to improve the adjustment technique of the SSS-T method and the accuracy of MinB to increase coincidence rates between proper sleep posture and sleep position.

5.7 Effect on Pillow Adjustment for Straight Neck

5.7.1 Introduction

Recently, many studies have reported that straight neck has no relationship with cervical pains. We have investigated the relationship between cervical spine alignment and chronic neck pain and shoulder stiffness with somatic symptoms, as well as cervical spine alignment and improvement of neck pain, shoulder stiffness, and somatic symptoms by using a pillow, for postural management at night.

5.7.2 Subjects and Methods

Eighty-three patients (25 males and 58 females, mean age 50.1 years) with moderate or severe symptoms (mean disease duration 105 months) who scored 8 or more points on the Somatic Symptom Scale 8 (SSS-8) were included in the study. The posterior tangent technique was used to classify the patients into 3 sub-groups: kyphosis group (L) ($n = 43$), straight group (S) ($n = 21$), and kyphosis group (K) ($n = 19$) (Fig. 5.28) Pillow height was determined using the SSS method, with a cervical tilt angle of approximately 15° in the supine position, symmetry of the head and neck in the lateral position, and smoothness in turning over in bed. The NRS and SSS-8 were evaluated before and 2 weeks and 3 months after pillow use, and the relationship with cervical spine alignment was analyzed.

5.7.3 Results

The baseline means of NRS were 6.8 for L, 6.5 for S, and 7.4 for K, with no significant difference among them. The improvement rates of NRS were 22.7% for L, 27.9% for S, and 29.3% for K after 2 weeks, with no significant difference between L-S and L-K. After 3 months, 35.1% for L, 44.1% for S, and 46.8%for K, with no significant difference between L-S and L-K. The baseline means of SSS-8 were 13.5 for L, 13.1 for S, and 12.8 for K, with no significant difference among them. The improvement rates of SSS-8 were 23.7% for L, 32.2% for S, and 22.2% for K after 2 weeks, with no significant difference between L-S and L-K. After 3 months, 34.9% for L, 50.7% for S, and 36.2% for K, with significant difference between L and S ($P < 0.01$) but no significant difference between L and K (Fig. 5.29).

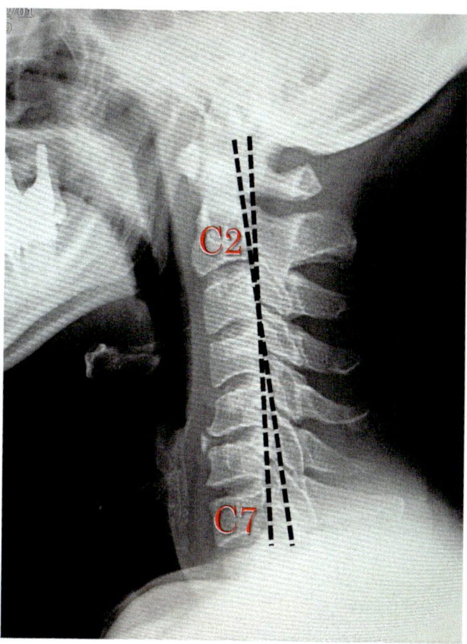

The posterior tangent technique is measurement of the angle of intersection of the tangents to the posterior surfaces of the C2 and C7 cervical vertebral bodies

Classification of cervical spine alignment (3 sub-groups)
Lordosis group (L): < -4
Straight group (S): -4 to +4
Kyphosis group (K): > +4

Fig. 5.28 Classification of cervical spine alignment using the posterior tangent technique

5.7.4 Discussion and Conclusion

Arguments on cervical spine kyphosis and prevalence began in the 1960s. In the early 1970s, D C Weir [3] investigated X-ray findings of cervical injuries and concluded that "Straightening or reversal of the cervical lordotic curve may be normal for the individual." D. Grob et al. [4] also concluded that structural abnormalities of the cervical spine in patients with cervical pain were coincidental and not necessarily the cause of pain. Roland D. et al. [5] stated that the proportions of lordosis and straightness were similar in symptomatic patients before cervical spine surgery. Kun Gao et al. [6] recruited young patients with cervical pain and abnormal cervical curvature, then evaluated the relationship between cervical lordosis and cervical disc herniation. The results showed that the degrees of cervical disc herniation and

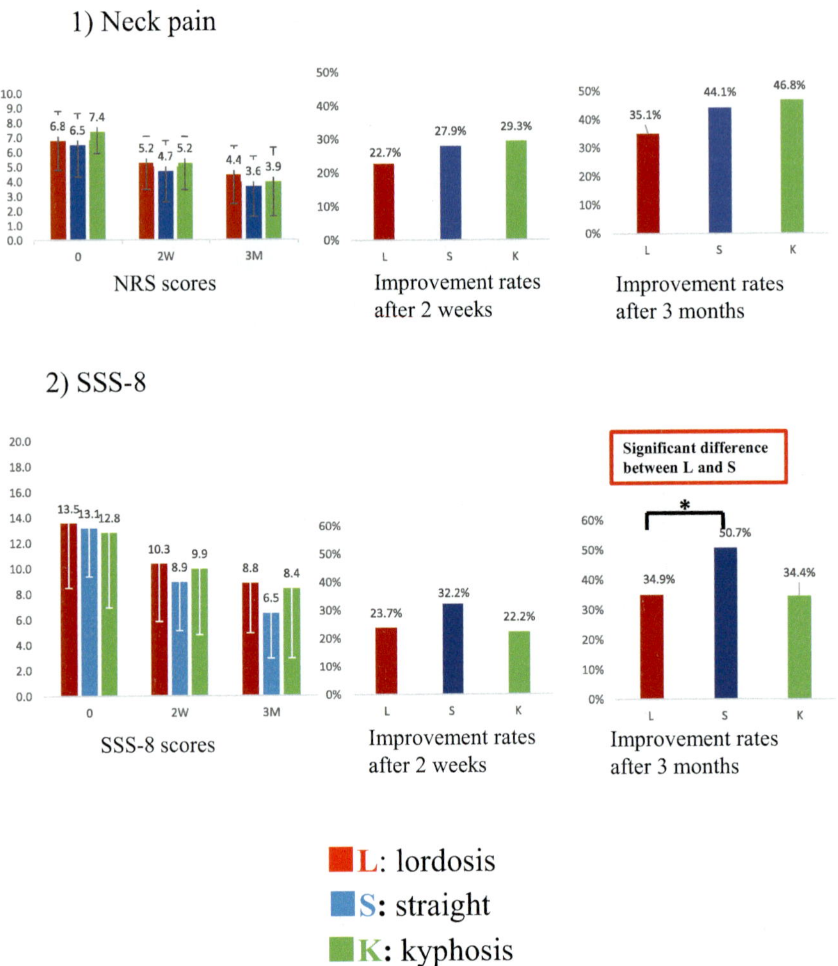

Fig. 5.29 NRS and SSS-8 scores and improvement ratios by cervical spine alignment

cervical spinal cord compression were inversely correlated with cervical lordosis in these patients. Laura Lippa et al. [7] reviewed articles published up to 2017 on the issues between cervical spine alignment and clinical symptoms and found majority of articles denying the relationship but a few affirming. They mentioned that it is essential to continue to study as many objective parameters as possible to correlate them with Health Related QOL measures.

We investigated the association between chronic neck pain and shoulder stiffness with somatic symptoms and cervical spine alignment. Many preceding studies were conducted in healthy volunteers or patients with mild pain (NRS score 3 or less). However, subjects (NRS mean score 6.9) in our study showed a high percentage of with S or K, means having abnormal alignments. As for the effect of pillow adjustment, pains and somatic symptoms before pillow use indicated no relationship with cervical spine alignment, and all symptoms improved by pillow adjustments, but the improvement rates of somatic symptoms were significantly higher in the straight group than in the Lordosis group.

5.8 Need for Pillow Adjustment for Patients with Rheumatoid Arthritis

Approximately 70% of patients with rheumatoid arthritis (RA) have cervical spine lesions, including axial subluxation and mid- and lower cervical lesions, and many patients complain of sleep disturbances due to cervical spine symptoms such as neck pain, numbness in the hands, and headache that prevent sound sleep. X-ray images (standing and supine) of spinal deformity in RA are shown in (Fig. 5.30), as are changes in cervical spine alignment in RA patients in the supine position without a pillow and with an optimal pillow (Fig. 5.31).

I collaborated with Professor Toru Suguro (now Professor Emeritus) of Toho University Sakura Hospital in his outpatient clinic specializing in RA from 2003 to 2009, on the optimal pillow for patients with RA.

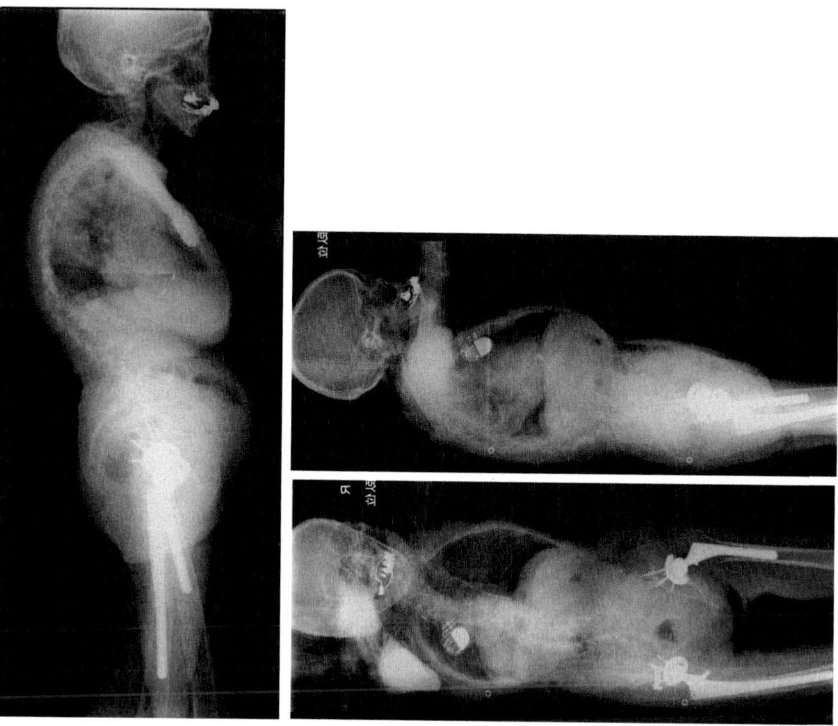

Fig. 5.30 Standing and supine positions in rheumatoid arthritis patients with spinal deformities

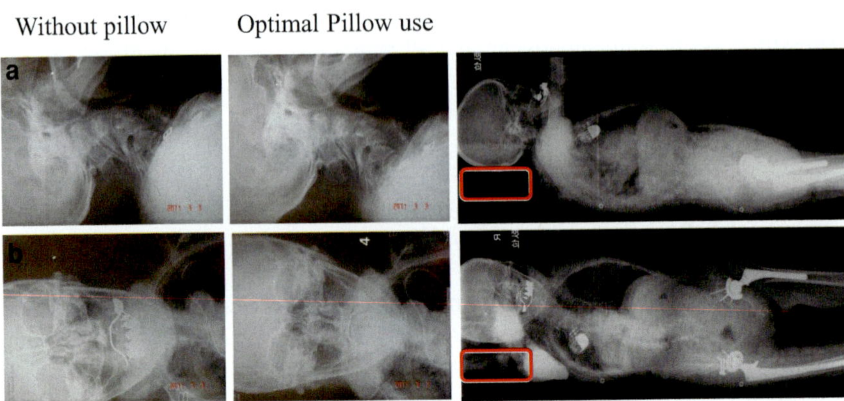

Fig. 5.31 Changes in cervical spine alignment without pillow and with optimal pillow use (neck and whole body) in patients with rheumatoid arthritis. (**a**) Sagittal plane (**b**) Coronal plane

Pillows for 43 RA patients, mean age 59.7 years, were adjusted using the SSS method (Fig. 5.1), and cervical symptoms and sleep were evaluated using the Pillow Score (PS) for RA*, VAS, and Face Scale. After follow-up period (mean duration 13.6 weeks), 93% of patients indicated that pillow adjustment facilitated turning overs, improved symptoms, and provided sound sleeps. Improvement rate of the PS for RA was 43.5%, particularly high improvement in ADL (52.6%) and satisfaction (69.0%). The cervical tilt angle in the supine position by the PS improvement was 14.6° in markedly improved 32 patients, 16.6° in improved 9 patients, 16.0° in 1 patient with no change, and 12.0° in deteriorated 1 patient, showing no correlation between symptom improvement and the supine cervical tilt angle. The ADI was 3.4 mm without a pillow, 3.7 mm with an optimal pillow, and with a too high pillow (optimal pillow plus 25 mm), with no significant differences. It was suggested that rests of cervical spine performed by optimal pillows during sleep may suppress inflammations of the spinal cord, nerve roots, and intervertebral joints in a relatively short period. In the middle-term observation for 2 years and over, it was suggested that cervical re-alignments were induced. The readjustment of pillow should be necessary conforming to this re-alignment.

*The Pillow Score (PS) (Fig. 5.32) was created by modifying The JOA score of the Japanese Orthopaedic Association (JOA). It is used to evaluate neck symptoms and general sleep symptoms, and to determine treatment outcomes. The PS is calculated by scoring subjective symptoms, objective findings, ADLs, and satisfaction on a 45-point scale. The Pillow Score for rheumatoid arthritis (PS for RA) (Fig. 5.33) was a modified version of PS with questions appropriate for RA.

In the past, RA patients' complains of neck pain and headache from the waking up time were interpreted as inevitable, as were joint pains. However, with the use of the optimal pillow, improvement in symptoms was observed after a short period of therapy. After middle-term follow-up for 6 years, the mean cervical tilt angle in the supine position was 8.1° before the pillow use, but after 3–12 repetitions of pillow adjustment, mean 6.8 times for 6 years, the mean angle became 13.3°, approaching that of normal subjects (15.2°) (Fig. 5.34). Conversely, during the 6 years after the

Pillow-based outcomes assessment measures :Pillow Score (PS)

name			date			date		
			before		score	after		score
1		subjective symptoms			score 9			score 9
A		About neck pain						
	a	No neck pain at all			3			3
	b	Occasional mild neck pain			2			2
	c	Constant or sometimes severe neck pain			1			1
	d	Constant severe neck pain			0			0
B		Upper limb pain and numbness						
	a	No upper limb pain or numbness at all			3			3
	b	Occasional mild upper limb pain and numbness			2			2
	c	Constant upper limb pain and numbness or sometimes severe upper limb pain and numbness			1			1
	d	Constant severe upper limb pain and numbness			0			0
C		Upper limb capability (manual tasks)						
	a	Totally normal daily life is possible.			3			3
	b	Able to carry out daily activities, but sometimes feels pain, numbness and weakness			2			2
	c	Slightly impaired in daily life with pain, numbness and weakness			1			1
	d	Extremely impaired in daily life with pain, numbness and weakness.			0			0
2		objective findings			score 10			score 10
A		Cervical spine ROM						
	a	Normal			2			2
	b	Light limitation			1			1
	c	Significant limitation			0			0
B		Jackson & Spurling test						
	a	Negative			2			2
	b	Scapular pain only			1			1
	c	Positive			0			0
C		Tenderness at Triger Point (scapula, upper limb)						
	a	Negative			2			2
	b	One positive			1			1
	c	Both positive			0			0
D		Sensory perception						
	a	Normal			2			2
	b	Slightly perceptually impaired			1			1
	c	Significant perceptual impairment			0			0
E		Muscle strength						
	a	Normal			2			2
	b	Slight muscle weakness			1			1
	c	Significant muscle weakness			0			0
3		Activities of daily living (ADL)			score 16			score 16
			None	Slightly	stronger	None	Slightly	stronger
	A	Discomfort on waking up (e.g. shoulder stiffness, headache, numbness in the hands)	2	1	0	2	1	0
	B	Frequent wrong sleeping patterns	2	1	0	2	1	0
	C	Back pain after long periods of time in the same position	2	1	0	2	1	0
	D	Trouble with driving.	2	1	0	2	1	0
	E	Shoulder stiffness, neck pain and discomfort when facing down (computer work, office work).	2	1	0	2	1	0
	F	Difficulty in lifting hands	2	1	0	2	1	0
	G	Insomnia, lack of sleep	2	1	0	2	1	0
	H	Difficulty of turning over in bed	2	1	0	2	1	0
4		Satisfaction (sleeping comfort)			score 2			score 2
	a	Satisfied			2			2
	b	Neither			1			1
	c	Dissatisfied			0			0
5		Other symptoms related to sleeping posture			total 8			total 8
			None	Slightly	stronger	None	Slightly	stronger
	A	Snoring	2	1	0	2	1	0
	B	Apnoea	2	1	0	2	1	0
	C	Low back pain	2	1	0	2	1	0
	D	Pain, numbness or coldness in the lower limbs	2	1	0	2	1	0
total score				total 45			total 45	

Fig. 5.32 Pillow score

Pillow-based outcomes assessment measures :Pillow Score (PS) for Rheumatoid arthritis(RA)

name			date			date		
			before		score	after		score
1		subjective symptoms			score 9			score 9
A		About neck pain						
	a	No neck pain at all			3			3
	b	Occasional mild neck pain			2			2
	c	Constant or sometimes severe neck pain			1			1
	d	Constant severe neck pain			0			0
B		Upper limb pain and numbness						
	a	No upper limb pain or numbness at all			3			3
	b	Occasional mild upper limb pain and numbness			2			2
	c	Constant upper limb pain and numbness or sometimes severe upper limb pain and numbness			1			1
	d	Constant severe upper limb pain and numbness			0			0
C		Upper limb capability (manual tasks)						
	a	Totally normal daily life is possible.			3			3
	b	Able to carry out daily activities, but sometimes feels pain, numbness and weakness			2			2
	c	Slightly impaired in daily life with pain, numbness and weakness			1			1
	d	Extremely impaired in daily life with pain, numbness and weakness.			0			0
2		objective findings			score 10			score 10
A		Cervical spine ROM						
	a	Normal			2			2
	b	Light limitation			1			1
	c	Significant limitation			0			0
B		Jackson & Spurling test						
	a	Negative			2			2
	b	Scapular pain only			1			1
	c	Positive			0			0
C		Tenderness at Triger Point (scapula, upper limb)						
	a	Negative			2			2
	b	One positive			1			1
	c	Both positive			0			0
D		Sensory perception						
	a	Normal			2			2
	b	Slightly perceptually impaired			1			1
	c	Significant perceptual impairment			0			0
E		Muscle strength						
	a	Normal			2			2
	b	Slight muscle weakness			1			1
	c	Significant muscle weakness			0			0
3		Activities of daily living (for Rheumatoid arthritis)			score 16			score 16
			None	Slightly	stronger	None	Slightly	stronger
	A	Morning stiffness around the neck	2	1	0	2	1	0
	B	Morning stiffness in the hands	2	1	0	2	1	0
	C	Discomfort on waking up (e.g. shoulder stiffness, headache, numbness in the hands)	2	1	0	2	1	0
	D	Frequent wrong sleep	2	1	0	2	1	0
	E	Shoulder stiffness, neck pain and mood discomfort in a facedown position (e.g. housework, office work)	2	1	0	2	1	0
	F	Dizziness and nausea	2	1	0	2	1	0
	G	Insomnia, lack of sleep well	2	1	0	2	1	0
	H	Difficulty to turn over in bed	2	1	0	2	1	0
4		Satisfaction (sleeping comfort)			score 2			score 2
	a	Satisfied			2			2
	b	Neither satisfied nor dissatisfied			1			1
	c	Dissatisfied			0			0
5		Other symptoms related to sleeping posture			score 8			score 8
			None	Slightly	stronger	None	Slightly	stronger
	A	Snoring	2	1	0	2	1	0
	B	Apnoea	2	1	0	2	1	0
	C	Back pain	2	1	0	2	1	0
	D	Pain, numbness or coldness in the lower limbs	2	1	0	2	1	0
total score				total 45			total 45	

Fig. 5.33 Pillow score for rheumatoid arthritis (PS for RA)

initial pillow adjustment, PS scores increased during an average of 6.8 times pillow adjustments attempts, but in patients whose number of adjustments decreased, PS scores decreased simultaneously (Fig. 5.35). We believe that RA patients need to have their pillows adjusted repeatedly while monitoring the progression of physical symptoms and spinal and joint deformities. We tried to determine factors that make pillow readjustment difficult, but the number of patients was limited and inconclusive. However, patients with high inflammation, mutilans type of RA, or postural abnormalities such as kyphosis had difficulty in turning over and determining the optimal pillow heights (Table 5.2). It is advisable to readjust the pillow height during the period of stable inflammation. Figure 5.36 shows the radiographic changes in the cervical spine of patients with RA before and after using the three different height pillows. The three pillow conditions were no pillow, optimal height pillow, and high pillow. The case shown in the center has used the optimal height pillow for 6 years and has been maintaining better cervical alignment. As a result, she has got ankylosis which is an anatomically good position. Dr. Suguro stated that it was ideal for patients with RA to have spontaneous cervical spine stability and ankylosis with long-term use of the optimal height pillow. This suggests that RA patients can safely and effectively adjust their pillows using the SSS method (Fig. 5.1). However, RA patients with elevated CRP levels and marked inflammation, or severe cervical instability sometimes immobilized their head and neck with sandbags to prevent turning over. In these special cases, it is better not to encourage turning over in some situations.

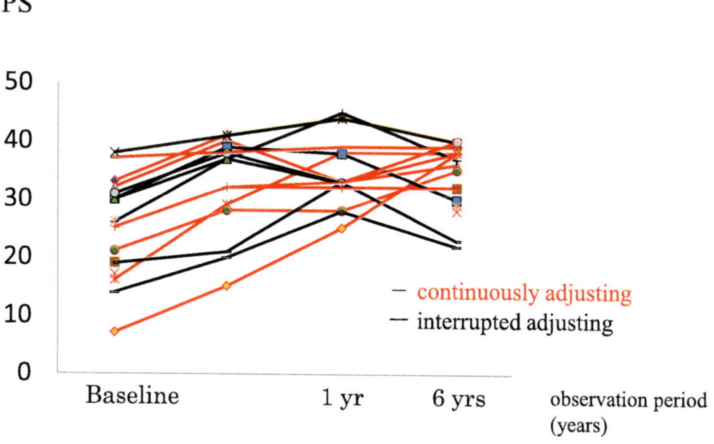

Fig. 5.34 Time course changes in the pillow scores in the supine position by pillow adjustments in patients with rheumatoid arthritis

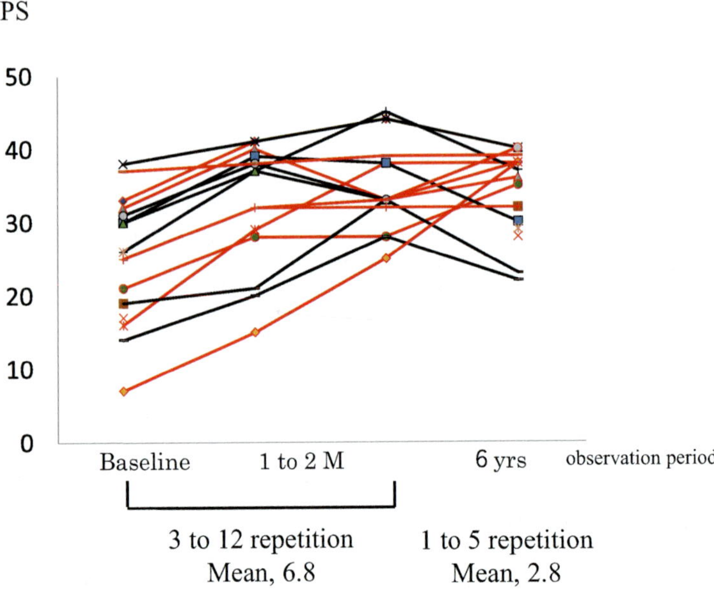

Fig. 5.35 Number of pillow adjustment repetitions and time course changes in the pillow score (PS) in patients with rheumatoid arthritis

Table 5.2 Suspected factors that make pillow adjustment difficult in patients with rheumatoid arthritis

Pillow adjustment	CRP	Biological medicines	No. of patients	Additional information
Optimal	Stable	In use	7	4 cases of kyphosis
		Not in use	4	2 cases of kyphosis
	Variable	In use	2	1 case of mutilans type and kyphosis, 1 case of kyphosis
		Not in use	3	2 case of mutilans type and kyphosis, 1 case of kyphosis
Poor	Stable	In use	1	Mutilans type
		Not in use	0	
	Variable	In use	1	Mutilans type and kyphosis
		Not in use	0	

Before pillow adjustment

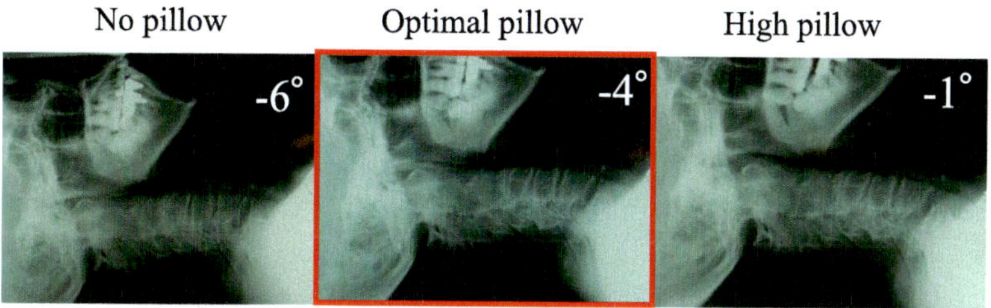

Middle and lower cervical spine unstable

Six years after pillow adjustment

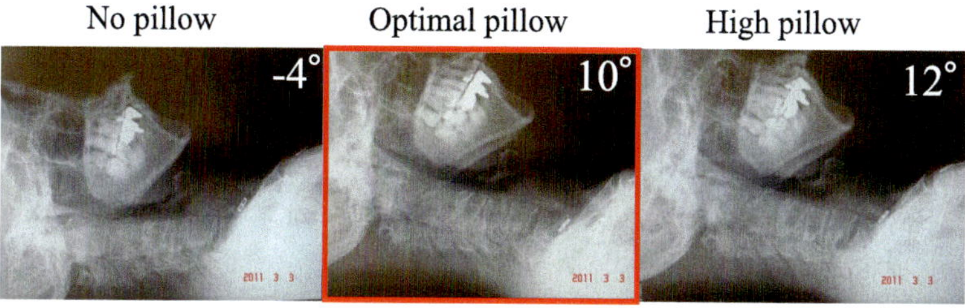

Better cervical alignment → Stable → Ankylosis in anatomical good position

Fig. 5.36 Radiographic changes in the cervical spine by pillow adjustment in a patient with rheumatoid arthritis

5.9 Need for Pillow Adjustment for Patients with Kyphosis

Age-related osteoporosis causes compression fractures, thoracolumbar spine spondylolisthesis, and deformity contracture of the shoulder and thorax, resulting in abnormal cervical spine curvature. Pillows in 15 patients out of 50 with constructed kyphosis with thoracolumbar compression fracture and 35 out of 50 patients with non-constructed kyphosis without compression fracture, total mean age 77.1 years, were adjusted using the SSS method (Fig. 5.1) and evaluated using changes of PS scores after a mean observation period of 23.4 weeks. The improvement rates were 55.7% for the overall score, 77.8% for subjective symptoms, 45.7% for objective findings, 55.1% for ADL, 92.3% for satisfactions, which were significantly improved ($P < 0.005$ each), in addition 92.9% for nocturnal symptoms, 91.9% for insomnia, and 49.7% for toilet frequency were also improved. When the pillow was adjusted for patients with kyphosis who had difficulty turning over, pain in several parts of the body and awakenings due to body movements during sleep were reduced in 90% and more of patients. The grand mean cervical tilt angle in the supine position when using the optimal pillows was 11.6°, 8.8° in

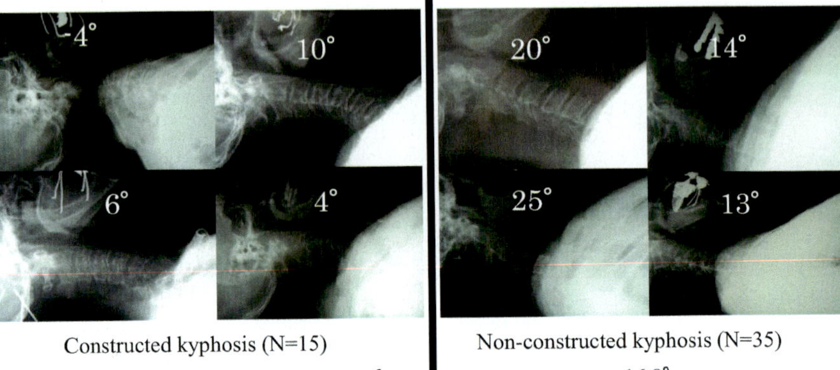

Fig. 5.37 X-ray of representative cases of constructed and non-constructed kyphosis. The mean of the cervical tilt angle is 8.8° of constructed kyphosis and 16.8° of non-constructed kyphosis in the supine position

patients with constructed kyphosis and 16.8° in patients with non-constructed kyphosis. The differences in supine cervical tilt angles between constructed and non-constructed kyphosis by X-ray are shown in Fig. 5.37. In comparison with 15.2° of mean cervical tilt angle in the supine position in non-kyphosis patients, these angles were lower in patients with constructed kyphosis and equal in patients with non-constructed kyphosis. MRI images also showed clear differences in cervical spine and cervical spinal cord alignment between constructed and non-constructed kyphosis. The angles of the two groups were negative in the no pillow condition and positive in the optimal pillow use (Fig. 5.38). Age-related spinal deformity can cause a variety of daily life problems such as gait disturbance, nocturnal back pain, and neck pain, and its involvement in locomotive syndrome and frailty syndrome, which have recently become problems in an aging society, is attracting attention. In patients with kyphosis, it is important to determine whether they have constructed or non-constructed one, and to encourage them to turn over in bed by adjusting strictly the pillow using the SSS method (Fig. 5.1), keeping in mind the cervical tilt angle in the supine position.

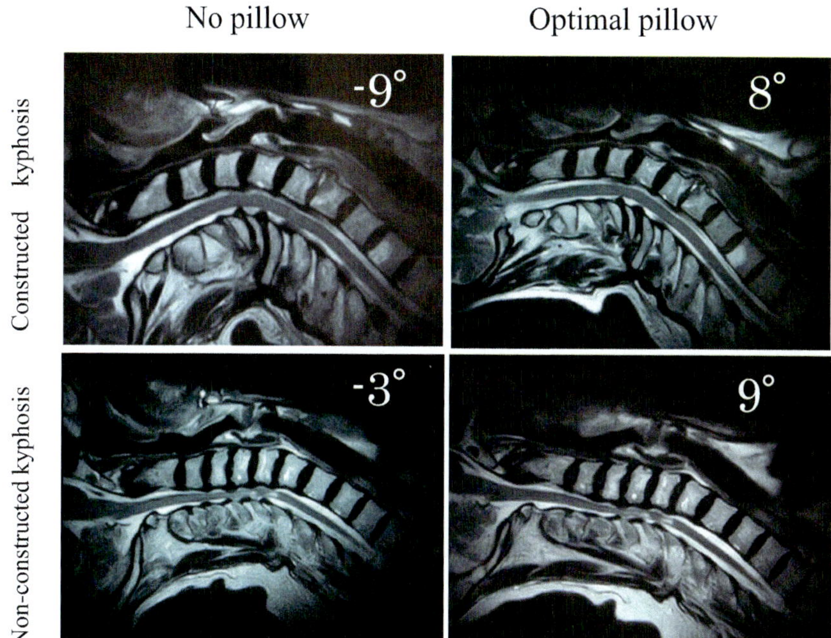

- In the no pillow condition, the cervical tilt angles in the supine position are negative.
- In the optimal pillow condition, the cervical tilt angles in the supine position are positive.

Fig. 5.38 The cervical tilt angles in constructed and non-constructed kyphosis by MRI

5.10 Effects on Pillow Adjustment for Patients with Whiplash Injury

The subjects were 25 patients with whiplash injury (acute and chronic) due to traffic accidents whose main complaints were neck pain and shoulder stiffness, mean age 45.2 years and mean follow-up 20.5 weeks. Mean PS score (Fig. 5.32) was 23.6 ± 7.2 points before pillow adjustment and 35.9 ± 6.6 points after pillow adjustment, with an improvement rate of 57.5%, including 62.8% for subjective symptoms, 42.1% for objective findings, and 64.2% for ADL. In particular, shoulder stiffness was improved in 64.6%, 78.2% for shoulder stiffness upon waking, and 48.1% for shoulder stiffness during the most burdensome turning the head down during the day. A total of 96.0% of the patients were aware that turning over in bed became easier or pain at turning over disappeared after SSS (Fig. 5.1), and sleep satisfaction increased by 74.1%. Sleep satisfaction increased by 74.1%. The supine cervical tilt angle using the optimal pillow was 13.8°.

The neck to periscapular region, which produces shoulder stiffness, is anatomically unstable during standing. Only in the supine position can be secured in which the cervical spine is not subjected to the weight of the skull, 4–8 kg in average, and does not require the support of musculoskeletal and ligamentous groups in the same region, but there are no guidelines for the sleeping posture. Symptomatic shoulder stiffness should be diagnosed and treated causal diseases appropriately, while non-symptomatic shoulder stiffness should be treated with daily lifestyle guidance, anti-inflammatory drugs, heat and exercise therapy, local injections, etc. Although improvement of poor posture is needed for shoulder stiffness as part of daily lifestyle guidance, no detailed information on the improvement of posture during sleep was available.

The most common pillow material used by 3670 patients who visited our Pillow Clinic from 2003 to 2006 was low-resilience urethane contour pillow (24%), followed by down (20%), buckwheat hull (18%), and plastic chips (17%). All of these materials are soft and easily deformable, making it difficult to maintain cervical spine stability and smooth turning over. Especially during the inflammatory phase in whiplash injury, when a patient turns over on a contour, soft, and ill-fitting height pillow, muscles including the sprained sternocleidomastoid muscle are hyperextended and pain occurs. It is important to select proper firm material and adjusted height pillow to stabilize the cervical spine while dynamically turning over smoothly.

5.11 Effects on Pillow Adjustment for Patients with Sleep Apnea Syndrome

For the treatment of obstructive sleep apnea syndrome (SAS), continuous positive airway pressure (CPAP) therapy is indicated for patients with moderate to severe SAS whose polysomnography (PSG) result is Apnea Hypopnea Index (AHI) ≥20. For patients with mild-to-moderate disease, treatment may include weight loss, mouthpiece, nasal tube, positional therapy, and otolaryngologic surgery (Fig. 5.39).

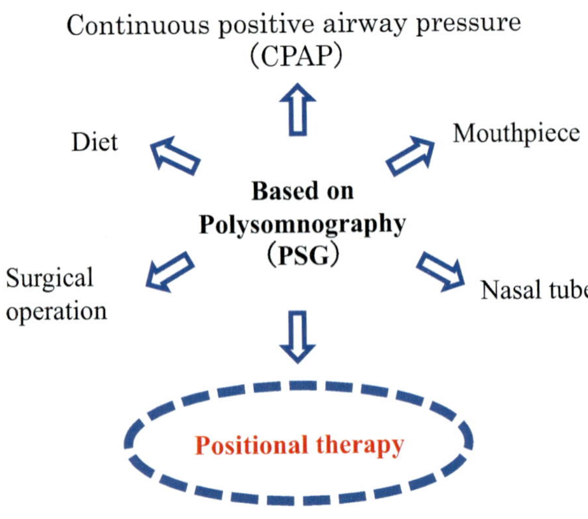

Fig. 5.39 Therapy of sleep apnea syndrome (SAS) after polysomnography (PSG)

Positional therapy is a treatment in which patients with SAS are recommended to sleep in the lateral position. In 2013, Akshay Menon and Manoj Kumar [8] conducted a systematic review on body postures affecting the severity of SAS, collecting reports published from 1983 to 2008. Eleven reports out of the 13 eligible ones concluded that supine sleep posture was associated with a severer SAS index in adults. P R Srijithesh et al. [9] compared the validated treatment, CPAP against the positional therapy (to keep people sleeping on their side) in the treatment of obstructive sleep apnea, because the positional therapy was less invasive and therefore expected to have better adherence. In conclusion, the positional therapy was less effective than CPAP to reduce AHI. However, it was shown to be better than inactive control on AHI and the Epworth Sleepiness Scale (ESS).

Currently, majority of researchers for sleeping believe that patients with SAS have a lower AHI when they sleep in the lateral position than in the supine position. However, in almost all reports, there is no prescription for pillows used during sleep. If all subjects had participated in the study using the optimal pillows, the study results should had been different. In other words, the AHI could be reduced also in the supine position if individual subjects used pillows that suited their physique, rather than forcing them to lie on their side with no pillow criteria. Let's imagine a patient with SAS who is admitted to the sleep clinic for the first night of PSG. We show the differences in three sleep postures (supine and lateral position) when the patient does not use a pillow, when a commercially available pillow, and when an optimal pillow adapted to the individual's physique is used in hospital room (Fig. 5.40). Therefore, we observed whether adjusting the pillow height and adjusting the cervical alignment in the supine position to secure the airway improves apnea levels.

We can present the following two studies:

1. A total of 8 patients, 3 women and 5 men, mean age 41.2 years, who were admitted to the sleep clinic for the first night of PSG were included in the study. Sleep duration in each position and AHI in the supine position were observed. Results showed that adjusting the pillow to the optimal height increased supine sleep time in 6 (80%) patients out of the 8. Mean supine durations in all 8 patients were 81.2 min with the inappropriate pillows and 164.4 min with the appropriate pillows (the optimal height pillow). Five (83.3%) out of the eight patients had a decrease in AHI even in supine position (Fig. 5.41). The results suggested that adjusting the pillow to the optimal height prolongs the supine time but does not necessarily increase the frequency of AHI.
2. AHI, minimum SaO_2, and stage changes were observed in 22 patients, 2 women and 20 men, mean age of 42 years, who underwent the first night. AHI improved in 19 (86.4%) out of 22. The mean AHI was 40.5 times/day in contour pillows, but significantly decreased at 31.6 times/day in optimal height pillows ($P = 0.044$). The improvement rates were 63.9% in maximum and 33.0% in mean. Eleven (50%) out of 22 patients increased minimum SaO_2 when changing the contour pillow to the optimal height pillow, but the mean change was slight, from

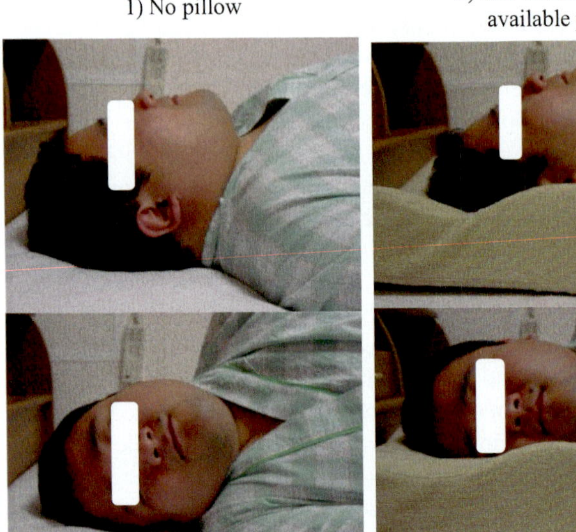

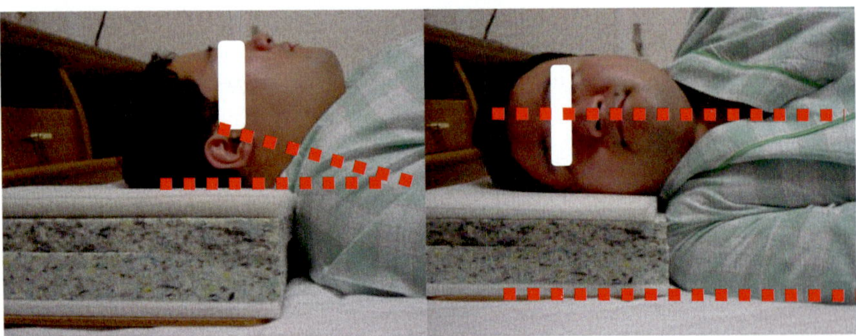

Fig. 5.40 Sleep postures of SAS patients under different pillow conditions (supine and lateral positions)

79.1 mmHg to 79.3 mmHg ($P = 0.85$) (Fig. 5.42). Regarding stage change, changing the contour pillow to the optimal height pillow significantly increased rapid eye movement (REM) sleep, significantly decreased Stage 1 (the shallowest sleep), and increased Stage 2. (Fig. 5.43). No correlation was observed between the age and gender of the patients with improved AHI or those with worsened AHI. The improved patients had no complications of nasal disorders or enlarged

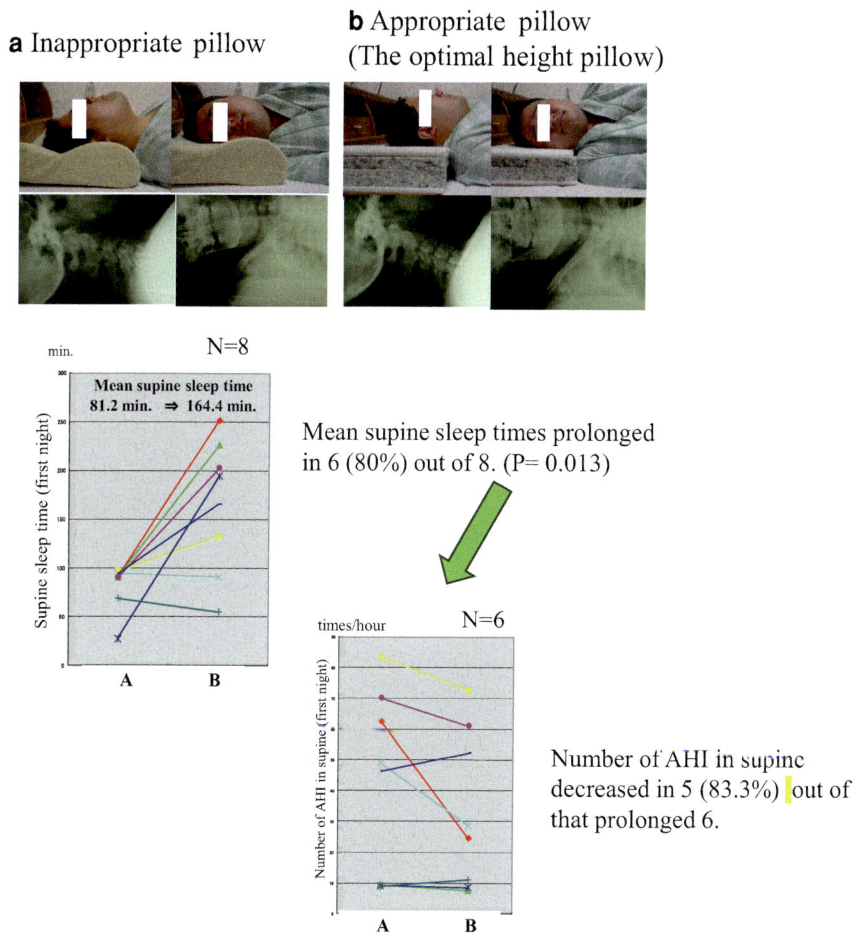

a Inappropriate pillow

b Appropriate pillow (The optimal height pillow)

N=8

Mean supine sleep time 81.2 min. ⇒ 164.4 min.

Supine sleep time (first night)

min.

A B

Mean supine sleep times prolonged in 6 (80%) out of 8. (P= 0.013)

N=6

times/hour

Number of AHI in supine (first night)

A B

Number of AHI in supine decreased in 5 (83.3%) out of that prolonged 6.

Fig. 5.41 Visual alignment and radiographs of the cervical spine when using an inappropriate pillow (**a**) and an appropriate pillow (the optimal height pillow) (**b**). Changes in supine sleep duration and apnea-hypopnea index (AHI) using the two types of pillows

tonsils, while the deteriorated ones had severe microtia, long face, and perennial allergies. The study suggested that proper pillow height adjustment tended to reduce the incidence of apnea in the supine position. The full physiological significance of REM sleep has not yet been elucidated. However, recent studies have suggested that REM sleep may be a measure of sleep quality. The implications of the significant increase in REM with the use of the optimal pillow will be unraveled in the future [10].

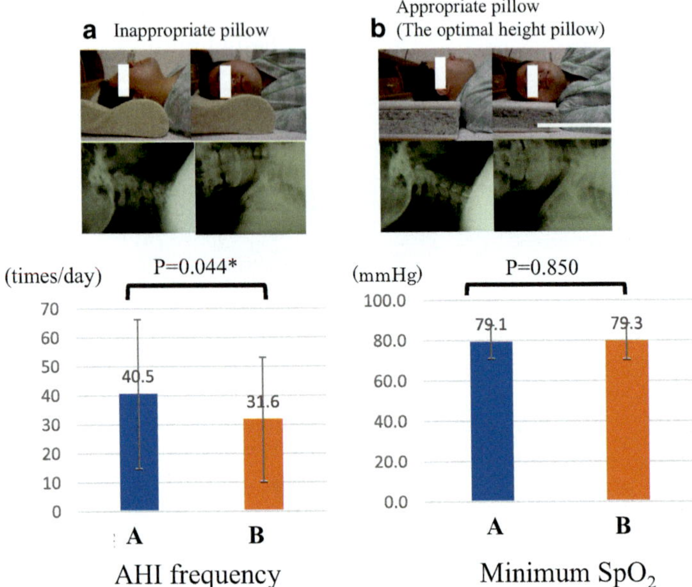

Fig. 5.42 Visual alignment and radiographs of the cervical spine when using an inappropriate pillow (**a**) and an appropriate pillow (the optimal height pillow) (**b**). Changes in sAHI and minimum SpO_2 in different pillows ($N = 22$) using the two types of pillows

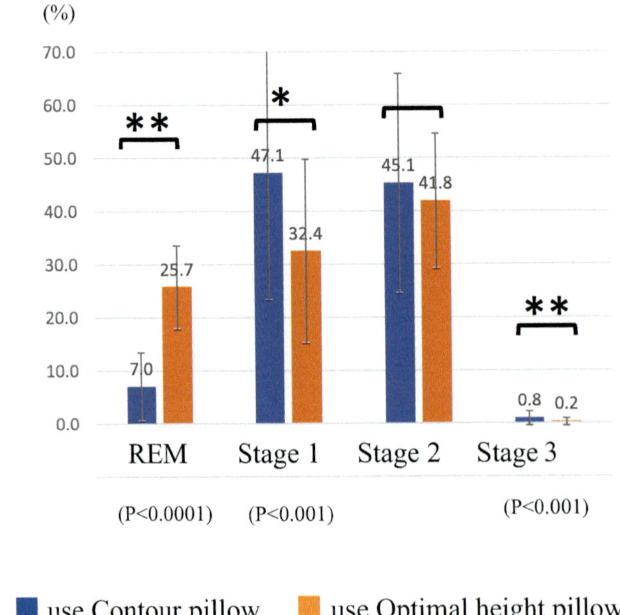

Fig. 5.43 Distributions of sleep stage in different pillows ($N = 22$)

5.12 Does a Baby Need Pillow Adjustment?

Any scientifically based answer has not yet been available to the question of at what age a baby or child needs a pillow. However, we have found a very interesting phenomenon that the body proportions of babies within 1 year of age, i.e., neonates or infants, were four heads tall (head length/height ratio), and the head circumference was larger than that of chest, so that the supine cervical tilt angle becomes optimal (about 15°) automatically without the use of pillow. We can prepare the X-ray images of elder and younger brothers as follows: they were male siblings who are 4 years and 3 months apart. Figure 5.44 shows the X-P lateral and supine positions of the older brother as a 0-year-old baby (11 months and 25 days). Figure 5.45 shows the X-P lateral and supine positions of the younger brother as 0-year-old baby (10 months and 25 days) (Figs. 5.44 and 5.45). In both brothers, the body axis

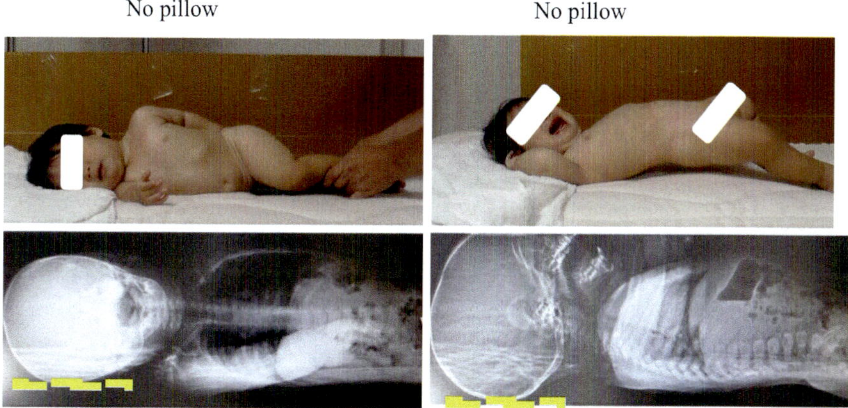

Fig. 5.44 Cervical tilt angle in the supine position 15.2° both in supine and lateral postures of a young child (older brother) without a pillow

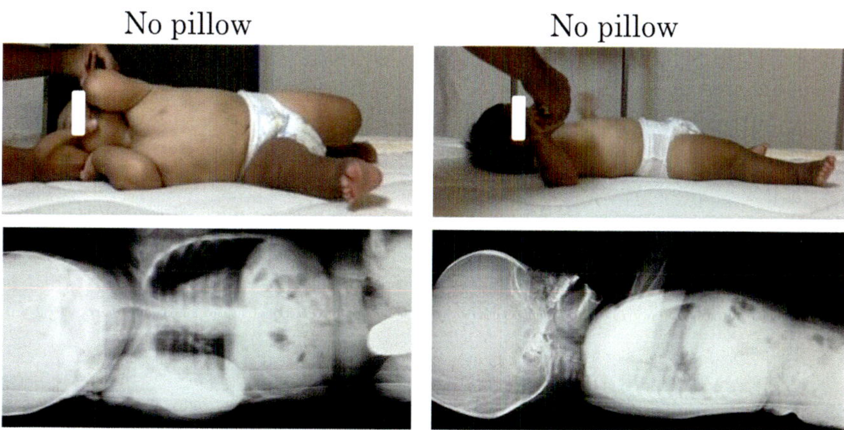

Fig. 5.45 Cervical tilt angle in the supine position 15.4°. Supine and lateral postures of a 0-year-old baby (younger brother) without a pillow

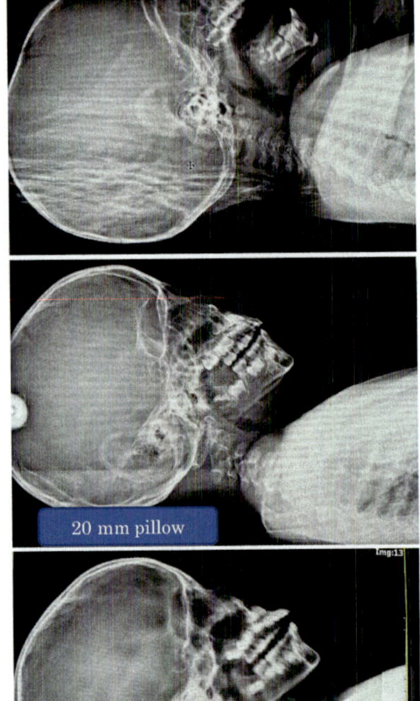

Fig. 5.46 Pillow height increased as he grow (older brother)

connecting the head, nose, and chest was parallel to the floor (symmetrical in the coronal plane) in the lateral position, and the supine cervical tilt angle was 15.2° and 15.4° in the supine position, which were very close to the optimal one in adults. Based on the result, 0-year-old babies may not require any pillows. Subsequent observations of optimal pillow height and changes in supine cervical tilt angle in the growth of the older brother indicate that the pillow height should be gradually increased from 3 years and 8 months to 8 years and 2 months. The clear difference can be observed comparing between 0-year-old babies and 8-year-old children, with the former not needing a pillow but the latter needing an optimal pillow (Fig. 5.46). At the same time measuring height of the pillow, we questioned about the ease of breathing in the supine position and the smoothness of turning over in bed, and we confirmed that even the child has made appropriate evaluations.

5.13 Cervical Symptoms and Efficacies of Pillow Adjustment in Children

5.13.1 Introduction

In recent years, children have been bending forward more and more in their daily lives, such as when studying, using smartphones or tablets, and playing video games. Similar to adults, many pediatric patients come to our clinic complaining of neck pain, shoulder stiffness, headache, and back pain. We observed the symptoms and characteristics of imaging findings of pediatric patients who came to our Pillow Clinic and investigated the results of pillow adjustment for postural management during sleep.

5.13.2 Subjects and Methods

Out of 432 children aged between 10 and 18 years at the time of their first visit to our clinic, 41 complained of cervical or spinal symptoms. After their pillow adjustments as part of the treatment, 12 (6–12 years of age range, 4 boys and 8 girls) had a good clinical course. In these 12 children, we conduct a retrospective study. A total of 9 children out of 12 had a history of attending other medical departments (e.g., pediatrics, otolaryngology, neurology, neurosurgery, and neurosurgery) for their chief complaints and concomitant symptoms. At the initial visit to our Pillow Clinic, the chief complaint, sleep-related symptoms, body size, and bedding environment were interviewed, and the imaging diagnosis, symptom course, and other special notes were recorded in the Data 5.1. Pillow adjustments were performed using the SSS method (Fig. 5.1) developed in our clinic. We prepared a pillow with a height that adapted to each patient's body physique and turning over in the supine position, using a handmade pillow (made of Japanese entrance mat and towelket) that was brought by subjects.

5.13.3 Results

The correlation coefficient between age and optimal pillow height was $R = 0.66$, indicating that the pillow height tended to increase with age. Nine (75%) out of 12 children showed findings other than physiological Lordosis (straight, kyphosis, disc instability) on X-ray. The clinical courses of patients showed improvement in headache, neck pain, sleep, dizziness, and so on. One child is presented here. An 11-year-old girl came to our Pillow Clinic complaining of neck pain and sleep disturbance. Her symptoms improved in the short term, but her cervical spine alignment (kyphosis) was unchanged at 1 and 5 years after treatment (Fig. 5.47).

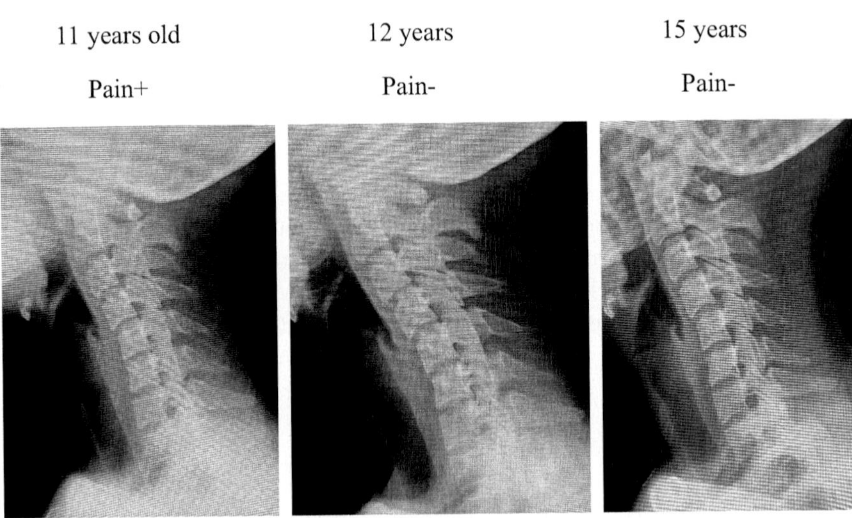

Fig. 5.47 Pain symptom resolved but cervical alignment did not change

5.13.4 Discussion

The optimal pillows were applied to children with symptoms of stiff shoulders and headaches in the study, and we observed markedly improved cases in some of the children. The majority of children showed poor cervical alignment in X-ray, but the relationship to the symptoms was unclear. Some of the patients had severe symptoms that restricted their daily life and prevented them from attending school, but even such children have improved. Considering the adverse drug reactions and/or systemic effects, we would like to minimize drug therapy, and noninvasive treatment is desirable. We believe pillow adjustment is one of the safe and simple noninvasive treatments.

Data 5.1 presents several cases in children in which symptoms improved with the use of an optimal pillow.

5.14 Survey on Body Physique and Optimum Pillow Height in Children

5.14.1 Introduction

Sleep for children is one of the important factors that affects not only their health but also many other aspects of their growth and development. We have shown the correlation between body physique and optimal pillow height in adults (Fig. 5.6), and the optimal pillow heights in children may also increase with their growth or body physique. However, few studies on the relationship between optimal pillow height and body physique in children were available. The purpose of this study was to investigate the correlation between body physique and optimal pillow heights in children.

5.14.2 Subjects and Methods

The subjects were 69 healthy children, 39 boys and 30 girls, aged 10–15 years, 15 aged 10, 10 aged 11, 14 aged 12, 15 aged 13, 8 aged 14, 7 aged 15, and mean age 12.2 years. After anthropometric measurements (height, weight, and shoulder width), the optimal pillow height was determined using the SSS method (Fig. 5.1). The pillow was made of three different types of materials, including low rebound urethane sheet, chip urethane sheet, and polyethylene sheet, and they were layered to create the pillow based on the determined heights (Fig. 5.48). Sheets for adjusting the height were given to the subjects, and they were instructed how to use the sheet for fine adjustment. The final pillow heights and usage conditions were recorded.

5.14.3 Results

The mean height, weight, shoulder width, and adjusted pillow height (mean ± SD) by age were as follows: in age 10 years, 137.1 cm, 33.2 kg, 35.7 cm, and 46.7 ± 6.0 mm; in age 11 years, 149.3 cm, 42.8 kg, 40 cm, and 55 ± 6.7 mm; in age 12 years, 152.3 cm, 41.2 kg, 40.3 cm, and 51.8 ± 5.9 mm; in age 13 years, 160.8 cm, 48.2 kg, 42.8 cm, and 57.3 ± 8.9 mm; in age 14 years, 161.5 cm, 54.3 kg, 43.4 cm, and 61.9 ± 5.0 mm; in age 15 years, 159 cm, 51.3 kg, 43.6 cm, and 60.7 ± 5.6 mm. The correlations between age, height, weight, and shoulder width and the adjusted pillow heights were R2 = 0.78, R2 = 0.84, R2 = 0.86, and R2 = 0.81, for aged 10 years, 11 years, 12 years, 13 years, 14 years, and 15 years, respectively. The post-use impression of the pillow was 26.8% for very satisfied, 40.8% for satisfied, 22.5% for neutral, 8.5% for dissatisfied, and 1.4% for very dissatisfied.

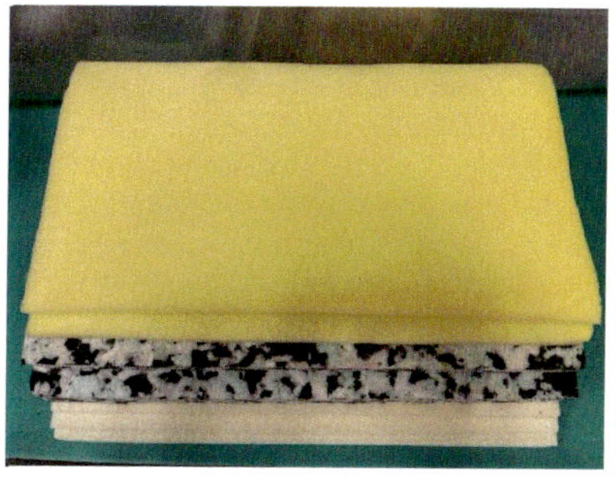

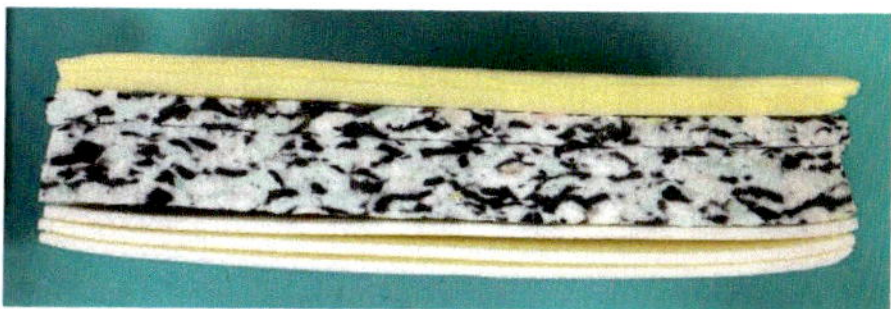

Upper layer：polyurethane sheet (soft)
Middle layer：chipped urethane sheet (medium firm)
lower layer：polyethylene sheet (firm)

Fig. 5.48 Handmade pillow used in the study

5.14.4 Discussion

All four parameters showed strong correlations with the optimal pillow height. It was suggested that children's' height, weight, and shoulder width increase with growth, and the optimal pillow heights increase simultaneously. The pillows materials used by the subjects before this study were 28.7% low resilience urethane, 23% down, 10.3% plastic chips, and 4.6% buckwheat hulls, which easily change shapes and heights, but about 70% of the subjects were satisfied after replacing pillows, suggesting that children also need to adjust their pillow heights according to age and body size growth. Therefore, we believe that it is necessary to adjust the height of pillows for children as their age and physique change.

References

1. Wong DW-C, Wang Y, Lin J, Tan Q, Chen TL-W, Zhang M, et al. Sleeping mattress determinants and evaluation: a biomechanical review and critique. PeerJ. 2019;7:e6364. https://doi.org/10.7717/peerj.6364.
2. Caussa JE, Cantarino CP, Tallon VB, Morera MAC, Escalera S, Sanchez D, et al. Automatic RBG-depth-pressure anthropometric analysis and individualised sleep solution prescription. J Med Eng Technol. 2017;41(6):486. https://doi.org/10.1080/03091902.2017.1350761.
3. Weir DC. Roentgenographic signs of cervical injury. Clin Orthop Relat Res. 1975;(109):9–17. https://doi.org/10.1097/00003086-197506000-00003.
4. Grob D, Frauenfelder H, Mannion AF. The association between cervical spine curvature and neck pain. Eur Spine J. 2007;16(5):669–78. https://doi.org/10.1007/s00586-006-0254-1. Epub 2006 Nov 18.
5. Donk RD, Fehlings MG, Verhagen WIM, Arnts H, Groenewoud H, Verbeek ALM, et al. An assessment of the most reliable method to estimate the sagittal alignment of the cervical spine: analysis of a prospective cohort of 138 cases. J Neurosurg Spine. 2017;26(5):572–6. https://doi.org/10.3171/2016.10.SPINE16632. Epub 2017 Mar 3.
6. Gao K, Zhang J, Lai J, Liu W, Lyu H, Wu Y, et al. Correlation between cervical lordosis and cervical disc herniation in young patients with neck pain. Medicine (Baltimore). 2019;98(31):e16545. https://doi.org/10.1097/MD.0000000000016545.
7. Lippa L, Lippa L, Cacciola F. Loss of cervical lordosis: what is the prognosis? J Craniovertebr Junction Spine. 2017;8(1):9–14. https://doi.org/10.4103/0974-8237.199877.
8. Menon A, Kumar M. Influence of body position on severity of obstructive sleep apnea: a systematic review. ISRN Otolaryngol. 2013;2013:670381. https://doi.org/10.1155/2013/670381.
9. Srijithesh PR, Aghoram R, Goel A, Dhanya J. Positional therapy for obstructive sleep apnoea. Cochrane Database Syst Rev. 2019;5(5):CD010990. https://doi.org/10.1002/14651858.CD010990.pub2.
10. Barbato G. REM sleep: an unknown indicator of sleep quality. Int J Environ Res Public Health. 2021;18(24):12976. https://doi.org/10.3390/ijerph182412976.

Q&A for the Pillow Clinic

6

Abstract

In this chapter, we have organized the frequently asked questions about pillows received at the Pillow Clinic and the replies. Some of the answers are based on our clinical experiences. Care was taken to keep the responses as simple as possible and easy for patients to understand. These sample Q&A will help you answer your patients' questions. However, healthcare and general market conditions may vary from country to country or region to region, so please use this information to tailor your answers to your specific situation.

Throughout this chapter, we have compiled answers to questions about improving daily life, such as neck pain, shoulder stiffness, depression, snoring, sleep apnea syndrome (SAS), and insomnia. Symptom relief, such as numbness, cervical disc herniation, lumber disc herniation, low back pain, rheumatoid arthritis, scoliosis, straight neck, headache, etc. are also included in this summary. Issues on sleeping posture, such as prone position, kyphosis, sleep position, lateral position, and turn over are also discussed. There are suggestions for pillow qualities such as commercially available pillow, pillow material, urethane pillow, polyurethane pillow, foam pillow, custom-made pillow, contour pillow, higher pillow, lower pillow, pillow size, pillow for children, without pillows, and beddings such as hard mattress, soft mattress, foam mattress, high density foam mattress, Japanese futon, comforter, pajamas, hag pillow, waterbed, smart pillow, smart Mattress are also reviewed.

6.1 Can a Good Pillow Help My Shoulder Stiffness?

Shoulder stiffness is divided into three categories by cause: intrinsic, symptomatic, and psychogenic. Intrinsic shoulder stiffness appears as symptoms triggered by common stresses in daily life, such as overwork, lack of exercise, fatigue, temperature

S. Yamada, *Orthopaedic Pillow*, https://doi.org/10.1007/978-981-99-0463-1_6

and pressure changes, lack of sleep, and poor posture. Symptomatic shoulder stiffness has symptoms as a part of disease. For example, in the field of orthopedics, osteoarthritis of the cervical spine, cervical disc herniation, cervical sprain, peri arthritis of the shoulder joint, and rotator cuff tear are causes of symptomatic shoulder stiffness. Other non-orthopedic diseases such as internal medicine, otolaryngology, ophthalmology, neurology, and dentistry are also causes of symptomatic shoulder stiffness as well. Examples include hypertension, heart disease, cerebral infarction, eye diseases that cause vision loss, sudden hearing loss, and temporomandibular joint disorder. Finally, psychogenic shoulder stiffness can be caused by psychosomatic disorders, depression, or mental illness. The first step in treating your shoulder stiffness is to know what is causing it. Once the cause is known, the issues that need to be addressed can be found, but this is not an easy task. It is also possible that a number of causes may be contributing to the onset of the condition.

If you're not sure where to start, let's start with the root of your shoulder stiffness treatment. That is "neck posture management." Postural management can be categorized by time of day: daytime and nighttime postural management of the neck. During the day, you can manage your posture with your own consciousness, but at night, or during sleep, you are unconscious, so your posture is determined by the bedding you lie on. In other words, a pillow not fitting the body physique can cause your shoulder stiffness, while a pillow fitting the body physique can relieve it. In many cases, not only shoulder stiffness but also autonomic nervous system symptoms associated with shoulder stiffness can be improved. Adjusting the height of the pillow to allow smooth turning over is thought to improve shoulder stiffness because it stabilizes the cervical spine while sleeping and puts less stress on the nerves, joints, and muscles of the neck. It is important to recognize that nighttime neck posture management is the infrastructure or foundation of shoulder stiffness treatment. If you ignore your sleeping posture, no amount of other advanced treatments during the day will improve it. You can start by managing your posture at night.

Note that if your symptoms do not improve after proper neck posture management, you may have symptomatic shoulder stiffness and should see an appropriate medical physician.

6.2 Can a Good Pillow Help My Depression?

Depression is not directly cured by a pillow, but patients with depression also need to adjust their pillows. The reason for this is that about 80% of patients with depression are said to be complicated by sleep disorders, and adjustments of pillow for sleep disorders and improvement of then may indirectly lead to remedy the depression. In our study, patients with chronic neck pain complicated with insomnia showed significant improvement in sleep disturbance after pillow adjustment. In many cases, depression can be alleviated by improving sleep posture, if the depression is simply due to prolonged sleep disturbance caused by poor sleep posture. Even for patients who have been diagnosed with depression, it is worthwhile to improve their sleep posture with an optimal pillow so that they can get a good night's sleep. We encourage you to adjust your pillow in conjunction with your medication.

6.3 Can Snoring Be Improved with a Good Pillow?

People sometimes think that if you sleep with a high pillow you snore, while if you sleep with a low pillow or no pillow you don't snore. However, no evidence has supported for this. It is true that a pillow that is too high or too low can obstruct the airway. We have revealed in many patients that their snoring improves when they use pillows with optimal height for their individual physique. If the pillow is just 5 mm too high or too low, it will not fit your body. In our questionnaire investigation of 40 people with BMI between 1 and 4, more than 70% of respondents experienced improvement in their snoring when using pillows with optimal height. In addition to helping to clear the airway, an optimal pillow height also relaxes the bones, muscles, and nerves in the neck area. To improve your snoring, start by sleeping on a pillow with proper height.

6.4 Can Sleep Apnea Be Improved with a Good Pillow?

Patients suspected of having sleep apnea syndrome (SAS), which is a recurrent attack of stopping breathing during sleep, are recommended to visit a sleep specialist. Polysomnography (PSG) is a comprehensive examination of the brain, breathing, blood circulation, and other functions during sleep. Patients who are diagnosed with SAS by PSG require the following treatments: lifestyle modifications (weight loss, smoking and/or alcohol cessations, etc.), mouthpiece or nasal tube fitting, or positional therapy. If the symptoms are moderate or severe, a treatment called nasal continuous positive airway pressure (CPAP) mask is used to widen the airway with constant air pressure to prevent airway obstruction. If the airway is narrowed by enlarged tonsils, surgery may be applied.

In addition, adjusting your pillow can also help improve sleep apnea.

In terms of our work with outpatient sleep specialists, I found two issues related to pillows in the testing and treatment of SAS.

First, the pillow used throughout the night when undergoing PSG has no standard. Regardless of a hospital pillow or patient's own pillow, it is not known whether the pillow fits patient's body or not. In other words, the test may be performed with an ill-fitting pillow. Second, the issues are treatment of SAS. As mentioned in Chap. 5, a part of treatment for SAS is positional therapy, which encourages patients with SAS to sleep in the lateral position. This may involve, for example, placing a tennis ball on the back to stop turning over, the use of a special pillow for the lateral position, or an alarm that starts vibrating when the patient is in the supine position. Many researchers on sleeping currently believe that SAS patients indicate a lower Apnea Hypopnea Index (AHI) when they sleep in the lateral position than in the supine position. However, we believe that adjusting the pillow can reduce the AHI in the supine position as well, rather than sleep in the lateral position using a special pillow. We strongly recommend that patients with mild-to-moderate SAS should try pillow adjustment first. In severe cases, CPAP can be used in combination with an optimal pillow.

6.5 Can Insomnia Be Improved with a Good Pillow?

Insomnia has a variety of symptoms and causes, and not all of them can be treated with a pillow. However, we believe that "pillow insomnia, " i. e., insomnia caused by ill-fitting pillows or poor sleep posture, is the most common type of transient insomnia. Also, even if the patient has other underlying causes, such as depression, poor sleep posture also occurs concomitantly with a high possibility. Therefore, I recommend that people suffering from insomnia should first adjust their pillow as a way to improve their sleep environment. If the cause of your insomnia is pain, such as neck pain or low back pain, note the following. In our research, we found not only chronic neck pain but also sleep disorders improved significantly from as short as 2 weeks after using the optimal pillow. Pain and sleep disturbance can become a vicious cycle when they become chronic. Continued pain causes sleep disturbance, and continued sleep disturbance increases sensitivity to pain. It is important to first try pillow adjustment that can be effective for both, then in combination with other treatments (medication, phototherapy, cognitive behavioral therapy, etc.).

6.6 Can a Good Pillow Help My Arm to Hand Numbness During Sleeping or Waking up?

Numbness of arms upon waking up could be due to poor neck posture during sleep. It frequently happens when the pillow height is not adequate. This is because when the cervical spine is flexed backward while sleeping, the roots of the cervical nerves are compressed, causing nerve root symptoms. When using the optimal pillow, you will notice an improvement in radiating pain and numbness in the upper extremities upon waking. Conversely, if you sleep in the same lateral position all night long, you will experience numbness and pain in your arms due to continued pressure on one part of your body. It is also important to be able to turn over smoothly in sleeping, which means being able to change position easily.

We recommend that orthopedic surgeons use pillows for patients with cervical spondylotic radiculopathy and monitor their effectiveness. This is because they can see and feel that many patients experience improvement in their symptoms in a very short period. According to Dr. Yasuhisa Tanaka, Director of Tohoku Central Hospital, who is the leading person to treat cervical spondylotic radiculopathy, he says that if there is no improvement after 3 months of strict pillow height adjustment and attempts at conservative therapy, surgery should be considered. This statement means that pillow adjustment is very important as a conservative therapy for the cervical spine. If you experience tingling in your arms and hands while sleeping or waking up, you should start by adjusting your pillow height and improving your neck posture. Of course, if adjusting the pillow does not improve, it may be caused by a variety of illnesses. We recommend that you see an orthopedic surgeon, neurosurgeon, or neurologist.

6.7 Can a Good Pillow Help My Lower Limb Pain or Back Pain During Sleeping or Waking

People experience pain in the lower extremities due to various reasons, such as foot pain, knee pain, ankle pain, lower limb neuralgia caused by lumbar spine disease, and so on. Depending on the cause, adjusting the pillow may or may not be helpful. If you experience knee pain, calf pain, or leg cramps during the night or upon waking, adjusting your sleep posture can help improve your lower extremity symptoms. Let's discuss leg pain, particularly knee pain and sciatica. Patients frequently complain of knee pains when getting up to go to the bathroom in the middle of the night, when turning over in bed, and when starting to walk upon waking. Sciatica occurs at similar times. In other words, the pain is felt when the hips and knees begin to move dynamically from a stationary position. The longer the knees and hips remain stationary, the more intense the pain. This means that it is important to be able to turn over and move around moderately with minimal energy while sleeping. Therefore, adjusting the height of your pillow to create a sleep environment that allows for easy turning over can help to alleviate some symptoms. Sleeping pain can decrease the quality of sleep and cause insomnia. In addition, insomnia can increase sensitivity to pain. This is a vicious cycle of pain. Patients diagnosed with knee osteoarthritis, lumbar osteoarthritis, or lumbar spinal stenosis often complain of knee pain and sciatica. These patients are often elderly and should avoid taking painkillers, especially NSAIDS before bedtime if possible. If you experience back to leg pain while sleeping or waking up, you may want to start with a relatively safe and noninvasive pillow adjustment and to use a medium-firm mattress to allow for smooth turning over.

Low back pain is also considered one of the main causes of poor sleep quality. Gianfilippo Caggiari et al. [1] conducted a systematic literature review of articles published until 2019, investigating the association of different mattresses with sleep quality and low back pain. Thirty-six high-quality articles were reviewed, including a randomized controlled trial (level of evidence I) by Kovacs et al. [2]. The results showed that a medium-firm mattress promotes comfort, The result showed that a medium-firm mattress promoted comfort, sleep quality, and spinal alignment. Firmness of mattresses was classified according to the European Committee for Standardization (2000). We also believe that the firmness of a mattress should be properly hard to allow smooth turning over. We recommend, for example, that you go to a bedding store and actually experience sleeping on the mattress you are considering.

6.8 Can an Optimal Pillow Improve a Cervical Herniation?

The optimal pillow does not cure a cervical disc herniation radically. But it can help relieve symptoms. There are three types of herniated discs depending on the area of the spine. When a disc in the cervical spine bulges and compresses a nerve, a person feels pain and numbness. Patients with a cervical disc herniation may find that using an optimal pillow may relieve pain in the supine position by stabilizing the cervical spine and providing a pathway for the nerves. Patients diagnosed with a cervical disc herniation can adjust the pillow using the SSS method (Fig. 6.1) in the same way as healthy individuals. Cervical postural management at night is especially important if the symptom is cervical radiculopathy, a radiating nerve pain, i.e., an electric shock from the neck to the hands. Conversely, symptoms are often exacerbated at night by an inappropriate pillow. Neuralgia can occur whether the pillow is 5 mm too high or too low in the lateral position. However, at the optimal height, there is a possibility that the painful symptoms may disappear.

Some people ask whether pillows are effective for cervical spondylotic myelopathy, which is a more serious disease. We would reply that the effectiveness of a

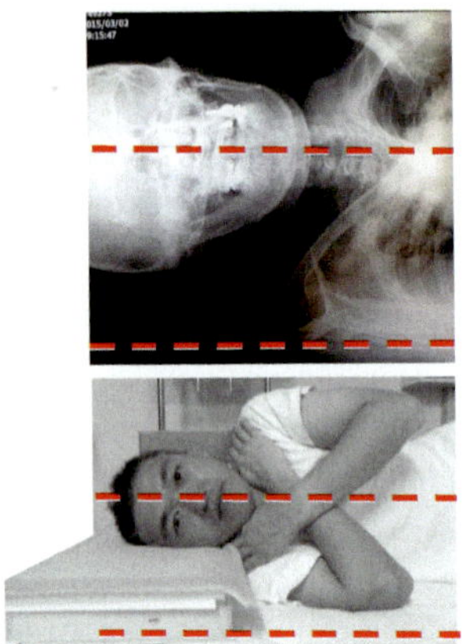

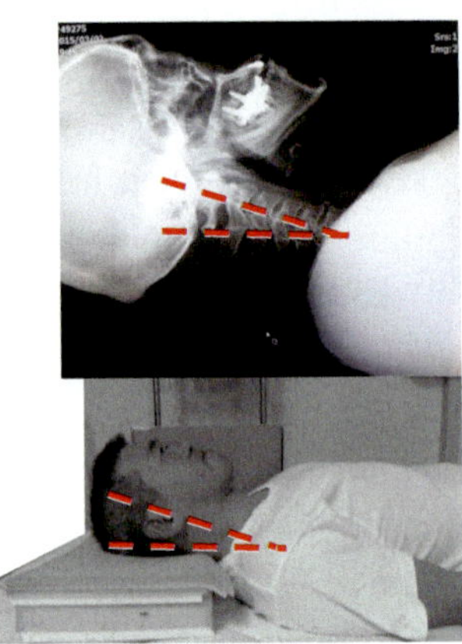

1st step: In the lateral position 2nd step: In the supine position

Set up for Spinal Sleep method (SSS method) is a method adjusting the height of -pillow for each person.

1st step: In the lateral position, the pillow height is adjusted so that the axis of head and trunk of the subject is aligned in parallel with the bed surface.

2nd step: In the supine position, the cervical spine is held at an angle of approximately 15 degrees anterior tilt from the bed surface.

3rd step: In the dynamic motion, we check how smoothly the subject is able to turn over according to the different height of pillow, adjusting increments and decrements of 5mm.

Finally, the pillow height that enables the subject to turn over most smoothly is the optimal adjusted pillow.

Fig. 6.1 Set up for Spinal Sleep Method® (SSS Method) (JP2004209099A)

pillow depends on the intensity of the disorder. If the patient develops sensory abnormalities in the upper extremities, motor paralysis, etc., then treatment according to orthopedic guidelines is the first priority. If you have numbness and weakness in both hands, but don't have muscle atrophy, then pillow adjustment can be effective for you. Using MRI, we have demonstrated that the spinal canal (anterior–posterior diameter of the subarachnoid space) in the sagittal plane is enlarged in patients using an optimal pillow. If you have been diagnosed with cervical disc herniation, you should first adjust the height of your pillow to improve your sleeping posture while sleeping. However, depending on the timing of the disease and the level of symptoms, this method may not be suitable. If your symptoms worsen or do not improve with the use of an adjusted pillow, you should see an orthopedic or spine surgeon.

6.9 Is Pillow Adjustment Effective for Rheumatoid Arthritis Patients?

Patients with rheumatoid arthritis are prone to deformity and dislocation of the spine, especially the cervical spine, and disc instability, making pillow adjustment more important than in healthy individuals. As the disease progresses and subluxation of the atlantoaxial joints and instability of the middle and lower cervical spine occur, it becomes even more important to control sleeping posture using the optimal pillow.

Patients with rheumatoid arthritis can also adjust their pillows safely and effectively using the SSS method (Fig. 6.1). It is said that more than 70% of rheumatoid arthritis patients have cervical spine lesions, and you may think that having neck pain and headache from the time you wake up is inevitable as well as joint pain. However, when using the optimal pillow, it is often possible to improve symptoms in a short period. The absence of pain at night also reduces the number of awakenings. In our study, after 6 years of middle-term follow-up, it was confirmed that even in patients with cervical spine instability on X-ray, continued use of the optimal pillow with repeated pillow adjustment may result in moderate stabilization of the neck bone alignment. In other words, for patients with rheumatoid arthritis, long-term use of the optimal pillow leads to both symptom control and a good prognosis.

6.10 I Have Been Diagnosed with Scoliosis. Do I Need to Adjust My Pillow?

Scoliosis can be divided into two main types, constructed and non-constructed scoliosis; constructed scoliosis is a kyphosis in which the spine is rotated (twisted) and can be idiopathic (no known cause), congenital or syndromic (neuromuscular diseases, Marfan syndrome, etc.). Non-constructed scoliosis is a functional or compensatory scoliosis that does not involve rotation and returns to normal when the cause is resolved. It can be due to leg length differences in the lower limbs or painful scoliosis (e.g., herniated lumbar disc). The classifications of scoliosis by age are school age, adolescence, adulthood, and senility (degenerative scoliosis). We have adjusted pillows for adolescent, adult, and senile scoliosis with good results whether the cause is symptomatic, idiopathic, or degenerative. The adjustment can be done by the SSS method, as in other diseases. In our experience, depending on the left-right curve of the scoliosis, some patients may have a difference in the smoothness of turning over from side to side, but in the end, it is important to determine the height at which turning over is most smooth after checking the entire right and left side of the patient. After using the optimal pillow, we often hear they find it easier to turn in their sleep, their neck and back tension has improved, and they are able to sleep better. If you have been diagnosed with scoliosis, the first step is to adjust the height of your pillow and your sleeping posture and reduce the strain on your spine when turning over in sleep.

6.11 Does a Good Pillow Correct Straight Neck?

Generally speaking, straight neck is a condition of the cervical vertebrae that is normally curved forward, is almost straight. It is said to be caused by prolonged use of computers or smartphones, which has become more common in recent years. Medically, the term "straight neck" is not clearly defined and not an orthopedic terminology. It is a term that probably began to be used in the realm of osteopathic and chiropractic therapy. In recent years, we have had many patients question of "Can the use of the proper pillow cure straight neck?" However, since we do not know if straight neck has any pathological significance in the first place, we cannot discuss the relationship with pillows. In the case of our Pillow Clinic, the radiographs of patients who complain of cervical symptoms are often "straight" before the use of the pillow, and even when the symptoms disappear after the use of the pillow, the patient neck is still straight. The standing cervical spine alignment before and after use of the optimal pillow is shown in Fig. 6.2. In other words, the symptoms such as neck pain and stiffness may have no relationship to straightness on X-ray. In the first place, the cervical spine alignment in the supine position with the optimal pillow is almost straight (Fig. 6.3). Therefore, we believe that straight neck is not related to symptoms.

In recent years, there are some papers in the world that straight neck and neck pain are not related. So if you have had chiropractic therapy or a massage and indicated that you have straight neck, we hardly say that this is the cause of your pain, stiffness, or other symptoms. What you want to improve should be your annoying neck pain, shoulder stiffness, and headaches, not straight neck. Regardless of whether you have straight neck on the X-ray or not, the optimal pillow will improve those symptoms.

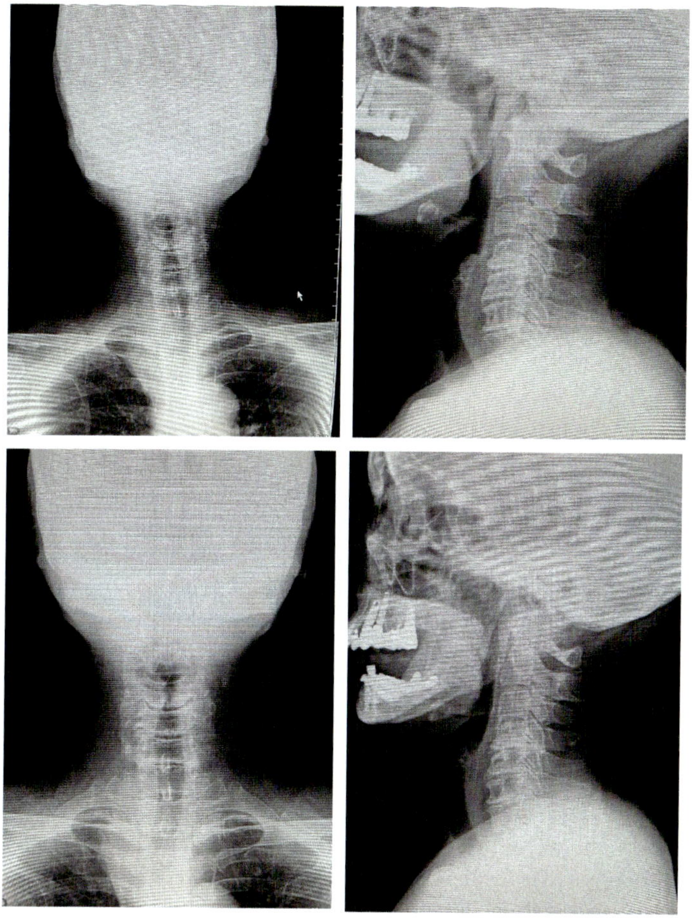

a

Pain+

b

Pain-

Fig. 6.2 Cervical spine alignment in standing position before and after use of the optimal pillow. (**a**) Before the pillow use (Pain +). (**b**) After the pillow use (Pain −)

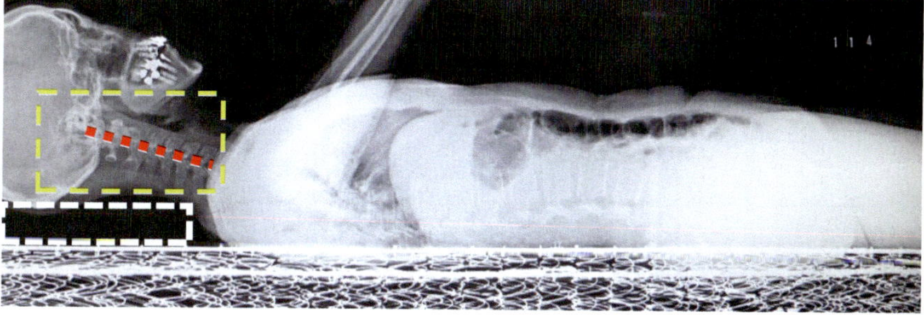

Cervical spine alignment in the supine position with the optimal pillow use is almost straight.

Fig. 6.3 Cervical alignment during optimal pillow use

6.12 Can Headaches Be Improved with a Good Pillow?

The best three most common headaches worldwide are migraine, tension-type headache (TTH), and substance abuse headache. In recent years, the personal, social, and economic burden of headache and its impact on global health disorders has become increasingly problematic. In 2007, Stovner et al. [3] reported that, globally, headache rates in adults were 46% for headache in general, 11% for migraine, 42% for TTH, and 3% for chronic daily headache. In 2018, Deanna Saylor et al. [4] stated in the Global Burden of Disease (GBD) 2010 that TTH was the second most common (22%) and migraine the third most common (15%) worldwide. In 2016, via the Diseases, Injuries, and Risk Factors (GBD) study [5], it was estimated that about three billion people were affected by TTH with 189 million and 104 million by migraine. From these figures, it can be inferred how headache is a major problem that needs to be solved.

In our Pillow Clinic, the cause of most of patients with TTH is a cervical spine, and most of them said "a strong stiff shoulder that developed into a headache" or " shoulder stiffness and headache developed at the same time." It can be caused by cervical spine conditions such as cervical deformity or herniated cervical discs, but it is also common in people who turn the head down at work (e.g., hairdressers, dental hygienists, or people who work long hours at the computer). The headache most likely to improve by a pillow adjustment is TTH. Another type of headache is "combined headache," complicating muscle tension headache and migraine. There are two patterns of symptom onset: tension headaches and migraines occur on different days, and tension headaches occur on a daily basis but migraines occur occasionally.

The three characteristics of migraine are (1) pulsating pain, (2) nausea and vomiting, and (3) aura (sensitivity to light, sound, and smell). The first choice of treatment for migraine is medication (Triptans, etc.), so we recommend that you visit an outpatient clinic specializing in headaches or a neurologist. However, before doing so, it is important to check if you are using an inappropriate pillow causing TTH during sleep. Improving TTH will eventually lead to a reduction in mixed headaches as a whole. In our pillow clinic, we frequently encounter patients who self-diagnosed migraine based on symptoms such as "pain on one side of my head" or "nausea." There are not so rare cases in which such patients are able to improve their symptoms by giving the pillow guidance. For all patients with TTH and migraines, we recommend that they first adjust their pillows to improve their sleep posture that is the infrastructure of their sleep.

6.13 I Have to Sleep in My Prone Position, Do I Still Need to Use a Pillow?

From an orthopedic point of view, the prone position is not a good sleep position for the cervical spine. People rotate the cervical spine to the right or left to avoid suffocation. Anatomically, the cervical intervertebral foramen is narrowed and the probability of nerve root symptoms increases. In addition, the patient may be awakened by large movements when changing from the prone to supine positions, which interrupts sleep. When we interviewed outpatients about their sleep posture, several common features can be found. They had used a variety of pillows, but nothing fits them, so before they know it, they've stopped using pillows and are sleeping on the prone position; or their shoulders had been compressed when they slept in the lateral position, so they have gradually gotten into the habit of sleeping on their stomach. Of course, these are not all the reasons why people sleep on the prone position, but these are the reasons we frequently hear in our clinical experiences. Conversely, if you encourage them correct pillow use and pillow adjustment, patients will no longer sleep on the prone position. From an orthopedic point of view, the prone position is not a good sleep position for the lumbar spine either.

The reason is that it causes pain due to the low back being inverted, forced into the same posture and it takes a lot of energy to turn over. It is more difficult to turn over in the prone position than in the supine position, as they have to lift yourself up and pull arms out from under them. This is thought to result in decreased sleep time and sleep quality. In conclusion, except for the special circumstances we describe below, you should try to avoid patient's prone sleeping by adjusting his/her pillow optimally.

Next, we can show the special situations in which the prone position is recommended. Dr. Shigeaki Hinohara, the late President of St. Luke's International Hospital, was the leading person to introduce American medicine to Japan and is the father of the term "lifestyle-related diseases." He advocated the Prone Positioning Method and developed his own pillow for the Prone Positioning Sleep. He passed away in 2017 at the age of 105, but it is said that he had been practicing prone sleeping for 5 h every night until then. We are negative about sleeping in the prone position all night, so I was interested in the prone position therapy recommended by him and the St. Luke's Hospital Prone Therapy Promotion Study Group, which is the opposite position to us. The prone position therapy they recommended for hospitalized patients was to use the prone posture only for short period, twice a day, not all night long. Originally, the purpose of the prone position was to drain vomit and secretions from the body and to secure the airway, but in Japan, studies were conducted since 1990s mainly by that study group from the unique perspective of preventing disuse syndrome in bedridden elderly patients.

There is another interesting report about the prone position. A new type of coronavirus infection (COVID-19) exploded across the world in 2020 and is still having a tremendous impact on society. In March 2020, The New York Times published an article titled "Low-Tech Way to Help Some COVID Patients: Flip Them Over," which showed a photograph of a COVID-19 patient at Rush University Medical Center in Chicago being treated with prone positioning. The effectiveness of prone positioning for Acute Respiratory Distress Syndrome (ARDS) had been validated before the COVID-19 outbreak [6]. After the pandemic outbreak, many evaluations of the efficacy of prone positioning in awake patients before as well as in intubated patients have been reported [7, 8]. In short, the appropriate sleep position must be selected according to the priority goals and circumstances.

6.14 Is the Appropriate Sleeping Posture the Same as the Standing Posture?

The optimal sleeping posture for humans has not yet been fully elucidated. The optimal sleep posture viewed from the front is symmetrical. Conversely, the optimal posture when viewed from the side has not yet been clarified. Therefore, the commonly accepted belief in TV commercials that "the sleeping posture should have the same S-curve as the standing posture" has no scientific evidence. In our research using X-rays, we found that the anterior curve of the cervical spine, the posterior curve of the thoracic spine, and the anterior curve of the lumbar spine all decrease significantly from the standing to the sitting positions, i.e., they approach straightness [6]. Therefore, the spine curve in the sleeping posture becomes different from that in the standing posture.

Another important aspect to consider is the curve of the neck when sleeping in the supine position (face up position). With an optimal pillow, the cervical vertebrae are nearly straight and slightly (around 15°) tilted forward when viewed from the side. Many people believe that because the neck is a forward curve in the standing position, it should be same in the sleeping position. However, this is incorrect. The reason for the curvature of the cervical spine in the standing posture is thought to distribute the weight load of the head on the neck due to gravity moving from the head to the tail. However, in the supine position, the direction of gravity differs and the cervical spine is not subjected to axial weight bearing, so they are no need for curvature. In recent years, contour pillows that follow the curve of the neck have become the megatrend. However, if the neck is straight while sleeping, we believe this "contour" is meaningless.

6.15 I Have a Round Back and Use a High Pillow. Is a Pillow That Fits My Supine Position Too High for My Lateral Position?

In kyphosis, where the back is rounded due to hunchback or age-related changes, sometimes the pillow is adjusted quite high in the supine position. Patients occasionally make questions, "Isn't that height of pillow too high, either face up position or side lying position? " This is not always the case.

For the elderly with round back, it is necessary to distinguish constructed from non-constructed ones. Non-constructed round back is a type of back that stretches when the patient is supine, and pillow adjustment is with no problem. Constructed round back is caused by a spinal fracture, spinal caries, or other disease that causes the spine to become stiff; therefore, the back does not extend when sleeping supine and the head does not attach to the pillow. In the latter type, as in the previous question, there is sometimes concern that the pillow height determined in the supine position might be too high in the lateral position. The human body has the ability to adapt, and patients with constructed round back also have become stiff shoulder joints and spines, so they need a high pillow even in the lateral position [8]. Of the approximately 60,000 patients whose pillows we have measured, only about five required definitely different pillow heights in the supine and lateral positions. We have therefore prepared two pillows for these patients, one for supine and another for lateral positions, and used them in the middle of the night. But they are exceptional cases.

6.16 I Always Sleep in the Right (Left) Side. Is There a Best Position for Each Person?

Several international papers on sleep posture have been published. Dr. Chris Idzikowski, the Edinburgh Sleep Centre, studied the sleep positions in 1000 people, classified them into 6 typical sleep positions, and examined the percentage of each sleep position. It is said he has concluded that there is a relationship between sleep positions and personalities. However, his paper does not browse currently and we can only glimpse it in the BBC report in 2003 [9].

Also, there is still poor scientific evidence on turning over, and almost no recent data has added to the knowledge of old textbooks. To begin with, no strict definitions of sleep position (supine, lateral, and prone) or turning over are present, and the difference between body movement and turning over is also not clear. The recommended positions are different according to the diseases, such as the left lateral position for heart disease, the lateral position for SAS, and the lateral position for low back pain, but the scientific evidence for this is insufficient yet.

We believe that there is no one best position for everyone, but that the important point is to be able to convert smoothly from any position to another with minimal energy. If you lie on your side all the time, blood vessels in some parts of your body will be compressed and blood circulation will be impaired. Shoulder joints are also compressed, resulting in high intra-articular pressure and pain. It is essential to adjust the height of the pillow and adjust the sleeping posture so that the patient can turn over smoothly while reducing local pressure.

6.17 Do I Need to Turn Over in Sleep?

Turning over is a human physiological phenomenon and is a must. If you don't turn over, there should be something wrong with your body or bedding. Turning over has many roles, including stimulating the circulation of fluids such as blood, lymph and joint fluids, regulating body temperature, and realigning the spine. The hypnology textbooks described that the average number of turning over in a night is about 20. In our laboratory experiment [7], the average number of it was 21.4 in the video analysis of the whole night, but some people turned extremely few (4 or 5 times), while others turned more than 30 times. Even patients who said they did not turn over themselves in their sleep, unconsciously did in their sleep was recorded in the video. The important thing is not the number of turning over, but whether you can turn over smoothly and without using force or waking up.

Many hypnologists consider turning over is a not good phenomenon that interrupts sleep. There is a test called polysomnography that monitors sleep depth and sleep quality. When turning over during sleep is observed using this test, arousal occurs at a time when sleep depth becomes shallow. However, our studies suggested that if patients use optimal height pillows, their sleep depth did not become shallow when they turned over. We need to change our way of thinking that we should keep the depth of sleep even during turning overs, rather than inhibiting turning overs that make the depth of sleep shallower.

6.18 What Is the Best Pillow on the Market?

In recent years, a lot of scientific researches on pillow design have been reported, and the pillow designs on the market have been influenced by the results of these researches more than a little. Pillow manufacturers have commercialized pillows that were invented by pillow researchers. Conversely, I think it is not few that researchers have chosen pillows for their studies without any clear standards and chosen one of the pillows on the market without any scientific basis. As a result, in the current market, the most common pillow shape is either a vertical or horizontal contour pillow, and the most common material is rubber, especially Latex (natural rubber), instead of conventionally used feathers. Currently, overseas products including pillows are being imported to Japan and overcrowded in the market. The probability that one pillow of them will fit each and every user's physique with different body shapes, ages, and gender by chance is never high.

Now to the question, "If I had to choose a pillow on the market, what kind of pillow would choose?" The answer is that you should abandon the idea of "choosing a pillow that looks good among pillows on the market." Pillow is the one that needs to be "adjusted" to fit your body. No matter what pillow you buy on the market, it will rarely fit you just right without adjustment. Furthermore, as you grow and age, you will need to change the height of pillow. It is impossible to use a pillow forever once purchased in terms of changes in physique. We recommend that you always have a handmade pillow that meets the three main requirements of a pillow: (1) height that fits your current physique, (2) firmness that does not sink more than 5 mm, and (3) a flat surface.

6.19 What Is the Best Material for the Pillow?

We can show some basic ideas regarding the choice of pillow material. The requirements of the material should be of a proper firmness suitable for turning over and adjustable in height. This assumes that you can adjust the height of the pillow yourself. The history of the pillow can be traced back as follows: when an Australopithecus fossil skull unearthed in South Africa in 1924 was found to have a crushed stone under it. It is unclear whether the crushed stone was used as a pillow or for ritual purposes. They generally said to be the oldest pillow, but unfortunately we have not been able to obtain any academic evidence to support this. In Japan, stone pillows began to be used from the Kofun period (around the third century).

After that, it seems that the pillow made by rush was used in the Heian period (around eighth century), and wooden pillows were used in the Edo period (seventeenth century onward). It means relatively hard pillow materials had been used. When we sleep, our anatomy requires that our head be lifted to a certain height. People may have known empirically that it is better to use a material with a certain firmness. Nowadays, new materials have been developed that feel good to the touch, retain and dissipate heat, and even space materials have been used for pillows and bedding. However, while these materials are pleasant to the touch, they are sometimes too soft for pillows and bedding and can compromise the most basic functions of supporting your sleeping posture and making it easier to turn over in your sleep.

When choosing a pillow material, it should satisfy the three most important requirements of the pillow in Sect. 4.2. The first and most important requirement is a material that allows you to strictly adjust the height. Once the height is determined, it must have the proper firmness to maintain it throughout the night. Second, the surface of the pillow does not need to be uneven, is flattened, to allow for smooth turning over. Finally, the height of the pillow needs to be adjustable according to changes in body physique and age. Considering the materials that satisfy these requirements, it becomes clear which materials are good or not. Beads, buckwheat hulls, straw chips and other granular materials, feathers and other soft materials, and low resilience urethane, which sinks over time, are not suitable. I have tried more than 20 different types of pillows, including ergonomic pillows developed overseas, low rebound contour pillows, and latex pillows, but my symptoms appeared from the time I woke up, or I was awakened in the middle of the night by pain, and I had to change to my optimal pillow.

6.20 Which Is Better, a Low Rebound or High Resilience Foam Pillow?

We are often asked questions such as "Is a low rebound pillow good for my neck?" or "How about a high resilience pillow?" First of all, let's clarify the definition of the terms "low rebound" and "high resilience."Low rebound (low rebound urethane foam in precise) is a urethane foam that suppresses "resilience" and increases "viscosity" and is defined as having a resilience modulus of less than 15% compared to general foam. Conversely, high resilience has no definition or numerical requirement. In the urethane foam industry, the opposite of low rebound foam is called "high resilience foam," which has more than 50% repulsive resilience and strong push-back force. Hardness does not mean high resilience. Even if urethane of the same hardness is used, "resilience"and "viscosity" differ from each other, and cushioning properties vary depending on the processing method. The important condition is that the material can maintain the optimum height for individual when you put your head on the pillow or when you turn over, that is, the height of the pillow does not change significantly more than 5 mm.

Some people feel comfortable with low rebound urethane foam pillows when they are used for a short time due to the pressure dispersion. However, as time passes after you fall asleep, your head will sink into the pillow and it will become difficult to turn over as if you were in a mold. A good pillow material is one that keeps your head from sinking into the pillow throughout the night and maintains the optimal height for easy turning over.

6.21 There Are Various Custom-Made Pillows, How Should I Choose One?

In recent years, we have often seen the term "custom-made pillow measurement and sales" in department stores and bedding specialty stores in Japan. The situation has changed drastically from when I developed the custom-made pillow in 2003. The "intended use" of a custom-made pillow and "what is to be personalized?" are different from each other. Our purpose is "to improve symptoms," and what we personalize is "the height of the pillow." This is because using a pillow adjusted to the optimum height will help you turn over smoothly and improve various symptoms during sleep and the quality of sleep. Conversely, the purpose of general marketed pillows is sensory, such as "good sleep" and "comfort," and "personal preference" is important. In other words, pillow makers do not adjust the "height" and "hardness" based on the customer's physique objectively, but complete custom-made pillows of various materials, heights, hardness, etc., by listening to "preferences" and "sensations." Even if those products have a catchphrase "born from medical research" or "supervised by a doctor," it is not clear whether the effect has been medically verified or not. Furthermore, it is questionable whether there is any real need for excessive decoration, such as making the shape more complicated or offering many kinds of materials to choose from, in order to increase the grade of the product and the sense of it being made to order.

There are many different types of custom-made pillows available, but you should always choose a pillow that meets the following three main requirements: adjustable height, proper firmness, and a flat surface.

6.22 Do I Need a Contour Pillow (Pillow with a Convex Shape Behind the Neck) to Support Your Neck?

Recent pillows with a convex shape behind the neck are designed to maintain a physiological lordosis (forward curve) in the supine position, just as same as in the standing position. However, it is unlikely that the convex shape of the pillows on the market will suit everyone's cervical lordosis. In our research, when a patient used an optimal pillow that improved the symptoms, his/her neck has been more like straight and not lordosis. In other words, you don't need a contour pillow that is high at the back of your neck and low at the top of your head.

The origin of the Contour Pillow (high fan shape at the back of the neck and low at the top of the head) can be traced back to research done in the USA in the 1940s on a pillow with a rolled pillow to support the back of the neck. The developer, Ruth Jackson MD. stated in her original book that the cervical roll pillow placed behind the neck would give the neck "a normal forward curve of the neck." Many researchers have then supported this interpretation, and it is thought that "during sleep, the cervical spine should be in a forward curve." But no clear medical evidence supports that a contour pillow was better than a regular-shaped pillow in terms of pain, neck disability, sleep pain, neck disability, and sleep quality. In fact, when we take X-ray or MRI of patients whose symptoms have improved with pillow height adjustment, the cervical spine approaches straight in the supine position rather than forward curve compared to the standing position. Conclusively, no reason is found to actively use a contour pillow.

6.23 Does a Contour Pillow Need High Sides and Low Center?

In addition to vertical contour pillows, pillows with horizontal contour shapes have also appeared in recent years. We often see such shapes in research papers overseas. This concept is based on the idea that the ends of the pillow should be as high as the width of your shoulders when you sleep in lateral position, and that the center of the pillow should be lower when you sleep in supine position because the rib cage is narrower than the width of your shoulders. However, for most pillow users of standard body physique, the human shoulder is flexible and shoulders and scapula are forward in lateral position, so the pillow height in the supine and lateral positions is considered to be approximately the same. Conversely, if the pillow is set too high in lateral position, it will require a lot of force to turn over to the side as if you were climbing a mountain path. As a result, it is not a good idea to make it difficult to turn over in sleeping. Therefore, a person of standard physique does not need a contour pillow that is high on both sides and low in the center.

However, this theory does not apply to people with exceptionally broad shoulders and a slender build. People with very broad shoulders will need a higher pillow in the lateral position. But at the same time, if you are thin, you may have thin back muscles and fat in the supine position, which can cause the appropriate pillow height to be too high in the lateral position. To deal with this, the idea of making the sides of the pillow higher and the center lower comes to mind, but our idea is different. Instead of making the pillow surface uneven, the surface of the sleeping surface (bed mattress, futon, etc.) should be made slightly softer to allow the shoulders to sink slightly when sleeping in the lateral position. Specifically, you should add a slightly softer mattress pad (5–10 mm) on top of the mattress or futon. This kind of device will make it easier to sleep in lateral position and turn over in sleep.

6.24 Which Is Better, a High or Low Pillow?

The argument which pillow is better higher or lower does not make sense. It is important to adjust the pillow to the appropriate height for each individual physique. The range of adjustment is strict and should be done in increments of 5 mm. If the pillow is 5 mm too high, the pillow user will experience neck pain, headaches, and numbness in the hands upon waking. However, it is not uncommon for the symptoms to improve as soon as the pillow is restored to its original height of 5 mm.

6.25 What Is the Ideal Pillow Size?

The height of the pillow is adjusted strictly according to the physique of the individual, but the width and depth of the pillow do not need to be adjusted as strictly as the height. A pillow 60 cm wide and 30 cm deep is suitable for people of standard physique, except for those with extra-large physiques (e.g., athletes) and special diseases (e.g., acromegaly). With this size, the user's head will not fall out of the pillow when they turn over in sleep. However, different races have different head sizes, shoulder widths, and chest thicknesses. Based on this standard for the Japanese, determine the size of the pillow based on your physique.

6.26 Do Children Need a Pillow? Are the Pillow Adjustments the Same for Adults and Children?

Children also need pillows. Strictly speaking, we think it may be necessary after the age of 1 year when standing gait begins. The basis for our assertion is that supine X-rays of infants under 1 year of age, before walking, show a supine cervical tilt angle of approximately 15° under pillowless conditions. This means that infants under 1 year of age can automatically maintain an optimal neck angle without the use of a pillow. However, the same infant's X-ray image taken after the age of 2 years did not show an appropriate supine cervical spine tilt angle of 15° without a pillow. This means that a pillow may be needed. Interestingly, a 2-year-old boy, for example, decided on his own that he felt comfortable it better when a pillow was made from a towel and placed under his head than when no pillow was provided. Subjective feeling and objective evaluation for the pillow were consistent. This phenomenon is not limited to this boy, most children also have a superior sensation that allows them to appropriately judge whether or not the pillow height is appropriate for them.

Currently, there is still no study on pillow with a certain level of evidence in children. We have applied the SSS method (Fig. 6.1) of pillow adjustment in adults and children aged 10 years and older. We could able to demonstrate that the method is safe and effective.

We guided children and their mothers how to make homemade pillows as shown in Chap. 5 and observe the time course of their symptoms. The method of adjusting pillows for children is basically the same as that for adults. It is important to keep in mind that the height and weight of children change drastically and the height of the pillow should change as the grows. The mother should observe the sleeping position of the child and if the child's head falls off the pillow, the pillow height is adjusted again, as the pillow height may have become too low for the child's increased height and weight. Parents should always continue to adjust the pillow height to suit the child's physique. At the very least, please never use pillows that are not adjustable, such as the contour low rebound pillows (children's pillows) that have become common in recent years, or traditional donut pillows.

6.27 May I Sleep Without a Pillow?

We have been questioned if you may sleep without a pillow. The answer is NO, except younger than 1-year-old babies. Since humans have shoulder width, a pillow is always necessary when sleeping in lateral position. In addition, in order to turn over smoothly that is a human physiological phenomenon, the entire body from the head needs to be one straight axis. Since the width of the head is smaller than the width of the shoulders, a pillow is essential to make up for this difference. Some people dislike pillows after purchasing a number of ill-fitting pillows. Such people need to have the idea of adjusting the pillow to themselves rather than not purchasing and using commercially available pillows.

6.28 Is it Better to Use a Hard or Soft Mattress?

Same as pillows, a mattress should ideally be adjusted to the firmness of the material to suit the individual physique and body part. Mattresses have a larger surface area than pillows, so their construction is more complex. Ideally, it should be able to be divided into several parts and the firmness adjusted according to each part of the body, such as supine and lateral sleep position, left-right difference of the body, etc. If the firmness cannot be adjusted so precisely, it should adjust it as much as possible. It is important to choose a mattress that matches your body size and weight as much as possible. Check mattress firmness for suitability in supine position. If there is a gap behind the waistline (near the fourth lumbar vertebra) where you can put your hand, it is probably too firm. Conversely, if the heaviest part of your body, from the hips to the buttocks, sinks into the mattress, then the mattress may be too soft.

The reply to the question of whether hard or soft mattress are better is "neither too hard nor too soft," but in the case of hard mattress, it can be adjusted by layering a thin soft mattress pad. But if it is too soft, it is difficult to adjust, so you need to pay close attention when you buy it.

We have developed MAKURAinBED® (MinB), which is a custom-made bed mattress completed by dividing the mattress into 12 parts and combining coil units of the hardness that matches each part of the body. The name "MAKURAinBED" is derived from the concept of integrating an optimal pillow and a mattress that fits

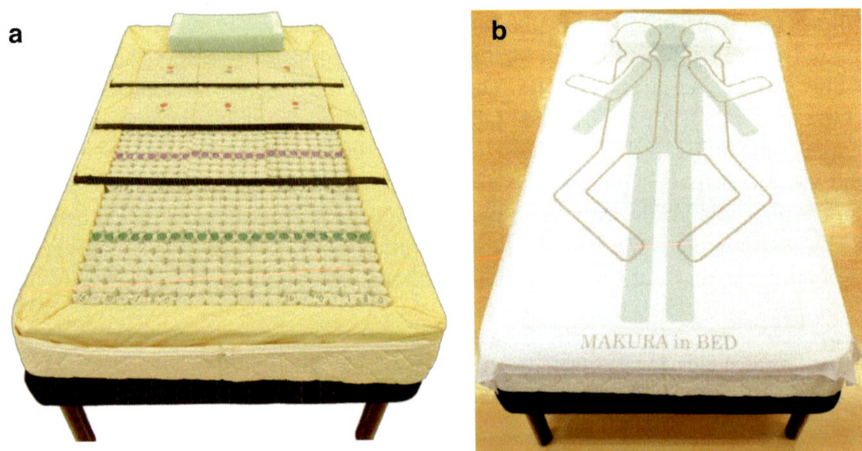

Fig. 6.4 Structure of the MAKURAinBED® (MinB) (JP201619726A) and the training sheet. (**a**) The mattress (12 coil units) adapted to each body part and the optimal pillow. (**b**) Covered with a training sheet for turning over

each part of the body. At the start of use, we recommend the sleepers to practice turning over in bed with a turning over training sheet over the coil unit. They will achieve the sleeping posture on the optimal firm coil unit (Fig. 6.4).

The reason for the development of this mattress is that we have experienced many times that no matter how strictly we adjust the pillow, the hardness of the pillow and the futon or mattress at home do not match, and the effect of the pillow cannot be fully exercised. In other words, the pillow and mattress should be considered as a single unit and adapted to the individual's whole body. Specifically, the MinB is a combination of 12 coil units with different spring multipliers of firmness in three vertical and four horizontal rows, which are customized to fit the patient's supine, lateral position, and turning over in bed. The combination of coil units can be changed as needed to accommodate changes in the mattress user's physique and symptoms. As a result of 5–10 years follow-up observations with adjusting mattress appropriately, many users showed improvement in neck and back symptoms. The result suggested that managing the sleep posture of the whole body was important.

6.29 What Type of Mattress Should I Choose?

Many different mattress materials and constructions have been marketed from many bed manufacturers. If the product name is the same, sometimes the mattress firmness is changed by the bed manufacturer according to the market preference or trend when revising the product. If you are considering buying a mattress, you should not choose it based on the manufacturer or the name of the product alone, you should go to a store or showroom and actually lie on the mattress and try it before making your choice. You should bring your optimal pillow and place it on the mattress and confirm whether you can turn over smoothly. It is important to note that if you only lie down for a very short time in a showroom, you will not be able to determine any discomfort or incompatibility with your neck or back, as you will not be able to get rid of all the muscle tension in your body.

You should try lying in at least one position, i.e., supine and lateral for at least 15 min each. As your muscles relax and your spinal alignment stabilizes, you can gradually be able to feel the difference between a mattress that fits or not. If you buy a too soft mattress, no way to adjust it afterward. Conversely, if you buy a little bit firm mattress, you can make some adjustments by putting a softer mattress pad on top of the mattress. Selecting the completely custom-made mattress is best, but even if you choose a mattress on the market, we strongly recommend that you choose a mattress with a moderate firmness that makes it easy to turn over in bed.

The main types of coil mattresses are "pocket coil" and "bonnell coil." Bonnell coils are not recommended because their surface support structure tends to cause the hips to bow or sink back. Pocket coils have a structure in which each coil is independent, contained in a non-woven fabric bag, so the heavy part of the back also sinks vertically to support the weight, and the surrounding coils have less affect. Be sure to choose one that is as durable as possible.

6.30 Which Is Better, a Low or High Resilience Elastic Mattresses?

Same as pillows, low rebound materials are not suitable for turning over in sleep. When the relatively heavy parts of the body, such as the pelvis and hips, sink in, it becomes difficult to turn over like a wheel stuck in a groove. Conversely, high resilience material has more supportive resilience than low one, but you need to make sure that your pelvis and hips do not sink in when you sleep for a long time and that you can smoothly turn over in bed. Compared to pillows, mattresses need to support heavier body parts (pelvis and hips), so it is necessary to select a mattress with moderate elasticity that can be easily turning over in bed according to individual weight and physique.

6.31 Which Is Better, a FUTON or a Mattress?

FUTON (Japanese matless) is a kind of bedding used in Japan since ancient times and is laid on tatami mats or the floor for sleeping. FUTON is made by side fabric and filling (padding), such as cotton, wool, down, or chemical fiber (polyester, etc.). In Europe and the USA, a futon is often referred to as a sofa bed. But sofa bed in Japan is used as a couch during the day and flattened as a bed at night, but is different from real FUTON.

In Western countries, mattresses are the most common type of rugs, made of a combination of coil springs and materials such as cotton, wool, foam, and latex. In recent years, mattresses made of only urethane foam or special resin fibers without springs have been on the rise.

Whether you are looking for a FUTON or a Western mattress, three functions are required: pressure dispersion, cushioning, and body temperature regulation. Pressure dispersion is to spread the weight of the body between the body and a hard sleeping surface so that the weight of the body is not concentrated in one point. The cushioning property moderately supports movement and turning over during sleep. The other is thermoregulation. In-bed temperature control is important and good deep body temperature control increases sleep depth. It doesn't matter if you choose a FUTON, mattress, or any other special bedding, as long as the rug serves these three purposes. Be sure to lie down on these beds and try the fit in the supine and lateral position and the smoothness of turning over before you choose the one that best fits your body.

6.32 Is a WaterBed Good?

There is a theory that human spine is in a near-optimal alignment when floating in water, and I actually bought a waterbed and used it for several years. In the supine position, the heavy pelvis and hips are supported by the moderate buoyancy, and in the lateral position, the protruding shoulders are comfortable without pressure as the water escapes to the surrounding area. I experienced that I can smoothly turn over in sleep with little effort. I use a waterbed containing only water, but various types of waterbeds have been on the market. Some are completely water-only and some have built-in fibers to adjust the firmness. However, there is no standard for how much water should be filled or what level of firmness should be chosen to suit an individual's physique. In other words, there is not enough medical and scientific evidence on how to use waterbeds. Additionally, some problems present. The total weight of a waterbed is 400–800 kg, which is 4–8 times heavy than that of normal wooden bed and mattress. Maintenance also requires expertise and special contractors. Also, depending on the user's constitution, seasickness-like symptoms may occur, so it is difficult to recommend it to everyone.

6.33 Can I Use a Hug Pillow?

When you use a hug pillow under your arms or legs when you sleep in lateral position, it distributes the weight and makes it easier to maintain a comfortable position. However, when the hug pillow occupies some part of the mattress, it becomes difficult to turn over resulting in the same sleeping position being maintained for a long time. Therefore, too much load is placed on one part of the body, causing neck pain, numbness in the arms and back pain upon waking up. In other words, it is not a good idea to use a hug pillow all night long.

One solution is not use it all night but at the onset of sleeping only. After that, it is best to choose something light and not large enough to be easily removed (kicked off) from the turning over space, after that. It is important for turning over, you do not place anything on your bed other than your own body, your pillow, and comforter.

6.34 What Kind of Comforter Is the Best?

When choosing a comforter or item to drape over your body, you should consider the material's heat retention (warmth), moisture absorption (ability to absorb sweat), moisture release (ability to dry sweat absorbed), and draping (fit to the body without leaving gaps).

Down, feathers, wool, cotton, and polyester as comforter materials have different properties. In terms of ease of turning over, feathers are the best. This is because it drapes well, yet is light and retains heat well. By adjusting the amount of down or feathers, you can use a thin layer even in the hot season. Wool is called a breathing fiber because it absorbs and releases moisture, making it an appropriate material for people who sweat a lot. It's a not good idea to use a blanket inside a comforter as a thermal barrier, as it clings to the body and interferes with turning over. It is better to put the blanket on top of the comforter. The blanket keeps the warmth between the comforter and your body from escaping. This way of covering is more effective at keeping you warm and allows you to turn over more easily. Conversely, it is difficult to choose a quilt for hot weather and places. Blankets are called "ket" for short, and we recommend summer blanket (towelket) or gauze-ket, which has excellent breathability, moisture absorption, and desorption properties, and linen, which feels cool to the touch and has a good tension and breathability. A half-size one (ca. 140 × 100 cm), which is half the size of a single blanket, is recommended. A "half-ket" is used with the arms and legs out and draped over the abdomen only, easier to dissipate heat and to turn over in bed.

Additionally, we recommend not using covers on FUTONs and blankets. The covers will cling to your torso and legs and make it difficult to turn over in sleep. If you are concerned about soiling your comforter without a cover, prepare made of washable material one.

6.35 What Kind of Pajamas Should I Wear?

There are three key requirements when choosing **pajamas**: material, shape, and size. The material of pajamas should be the one with low frictional resistance when in contact with the comforter or mattress, as not to disturb turning over in sleep. Cotton, silk, and recently developed functional polyester cotton are easy to slip and turn over. Conversely, raised fabrics and multiple layers make it difficult to turn over. From the viewpoint of the in-bed climate, it is necessary to select materials that match the air permeability, moisture absorption, moisture desorption, and heat retention properties. The basic shape pajamas (a combination of a top and bottom) make it easy to turn over in sleep.

The best **pajamas** are one that does not accumulate around the waist when the top is inserted into the bottom. Avoid fashions designed to look like a dress, as they will cling to your legs. Around the shoulders and knees, the ideal material and shape should be stretchable so that the joints can move easily when turning over in sleep. As a more detailed condition, avoid thick collars and hoods around the neck, as they can cause neck problems during sleep. Finally, regarding the size, in order to turn over smoothly in your sleep, the size should be appropriate, neither too large nor too small compared to your physique. In other words, you need to choose **pajamas** that allow you to "move" easily while you sleep. In essence, it is best to select a size that fits your body shape as much as possible after trying it on, just as you would select a size for suits or dresses these days.

6.36 Will There Be a Time in the Future When We Will Use Smart Pillow or Smart Mattress?

In the 2020s, the rapid development of Artificial Intelligence (AI), Internet of Things (IoT), Big data analysis, etc., will lead to the completion and use of Smart Pillow or Smart Mattress also in the healthcare field of sleeping. Many researchers are pioneering research and publishing papers on the issue. One of the reasons for the accelerated research is the belief that there are still many unexplored roles and effects of sleep, a human physiological phenomenon, and that its clarification and practical application will make a significant contribution to human health. Tsung-Te Chung et al. [10] evaluated the effect of the smart antisnore pillow (SAP) using polysomnography in patients with OSAS (obstructive sleep apnea syndrome) in a prospective, non-controlled, non-randomized, pilot study. As a result, the SAP is an effective positional therapy device for patients with OSAS of mild-to-moderate severity. Jin Zhang et al. [11] propose and implement a smartphone-based auto-adjustable pillow system to detect and treat sleep apnea. This pillow system can detect sleep apnea events in real-time using the blood oxygen sensor and automatically adjust to terminate the sleep apnea event. Songsheng Li and Christopher Chiu [12] developed the smart pillow to provide a relatively easy way to observe the user's sleep condition, employing a cloud-based health-sensing system is built in the pillow to collect and analyze data, help making decision of diagnoses, and treat some sleep-related symptoms. For the bed matless, Zicheng Zhang et al. [13] created a smart mattress consisting by 10 × 18 air packs containing a set of pressure and height sensors and two air valves and control units. The bed automatically perceives the user's body structure, body pressure matrix, and then automatically adjust to the optimal sleeping position and thereby achieve a uniform force distribution for a comfortable state. Furthermore, they predict that the smart mattress can connect to an auxiliary part of a smart ecosystem consisting of a smart pill box, a smart lighting system, and a microclimate system in the future.

These studies similarly aim for SMART CONTROL of sleep, but the parameters monitored are different from study to study. The most important parameter for us is the smoothness of turning over. We would like to develop a system that monitors the smoothness of static sleep postures (supine, lateral, and turning over) not only in patients but also in healthy people throughout the night and immediately gives feedback to correct pillow height and mattress firmness by remote control when a poor posture is detected. We want to create a social sleep infrastructure that allows anyone to sleep properly and safely anywhere in the world (Fig. 6.5). In the near future,

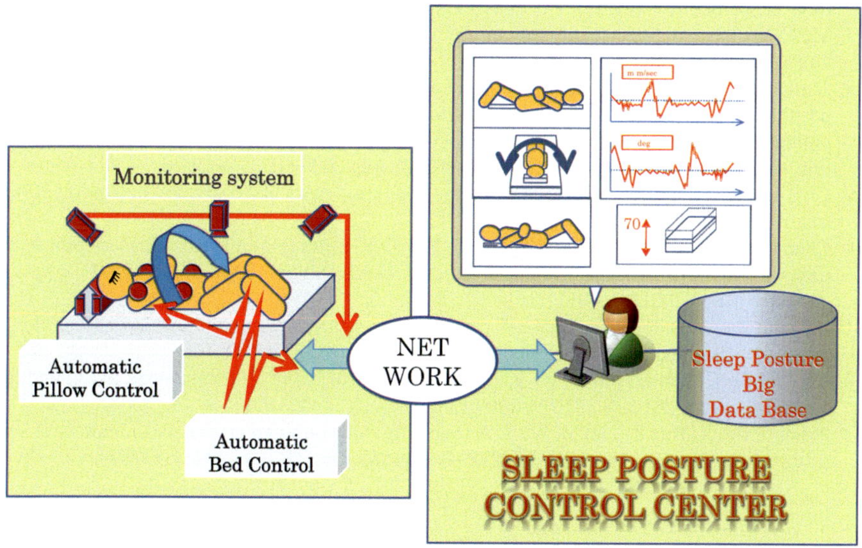

Fig. 6.5 Pillow and mattress system for monitoring and remotely controlling the sleep posture of all people, including patients automatically

the sleep environment, i.e., pillows, mattresses, and comforters, will be managed in an integrated system and will evolve into an AI (robot) that envelops humans and gives them good sleep and good health.

References

1. Caggiari G, Talesa GR, Toro G, Jannelli E, Monteleone G, Puddu L. What type of mattress should be chosen to avoid back pain and improve sleep quality? Review of the literature. J Orthop Traumatol. 2021;22(1):51. https://doi.org/10.1186/s10195-021-00616-5.
2. Kovacs FM, Abraira V, Peña A, Martín-Rodríguez JG, Sánchez-Vera M, et al. Effect of firmness of mattress on chronic non-specific low-back pain: randomised, double-blind, controlled, multicentre trial. Lancet. 2003;362(9396):1599–604. www.thelancet.com.
3. Stovner LJ, Hagen K, Jensen R, Katsarava Z, Lipton RB, Scher AI, et al. The global burden of headache: a documentation of headache prevalence and disability worldwide. Cephalalgia. 2007;27(3):193–210.
4. Saylor D, Steiner TJ. The global burden of headache. Semin Neurol. 2018;38(2):182–90. https://doi.org/10.1055/s-0038-1646946.
5. GBD 2016 Headache Collaborators. Global, regional, and national burden of migraine and tension-type headache, 1990–2016: a systematic analysis for the global burden of disease study 2016. Lancet Neurol. 2018;17(11):954–76. https://doi.org/10.1016/S1474-4422(18)30322-3.
6. Guérin C, Reignier J, Richard J-C, Beuret P, Gacouin A, Boulain T, PROSEVA Study Group, et al. Prone positioning in severe acute respiratory distress syndrome. N Engl J Med. 2013;368(23):2159–68. https://doi.org/10.1056/NEJMoa1214103.
7. Coppo A, Bellani G, Winterton D, Di Pierro M, Soria A, Faverio P, et al. Feasibility and physiological effects of prone positioning in non-intubated patients with acute respira-

tory failure due to COVID-19 (PRON-COVID): a prospective cohort study. Lancet Respir Med. 2020;8(8):765–74. https://doi.org/10.1016/S2213-2600(20)30268-X. Epub 2020 Jun 19.PMID: 32569585.

8. Ehrmann S, Li J, Ibarra-Estrada M, Perez Y, Pavlov I, McNicholas B, et al. Awake prone positioning for COVID-19 acute hypoxaemic respiratory failure: a randomised, controlled, multinational, open-label meta-trial. Lancet Respir Med. 2021;9(12):1387–95. https://doi.org/10.1016/S2213-2600(21)00356-8. Epub 2021 Aug 20.PMID: 34425070.
9. CBB news, sleep position gives personality clue. http://news.bbc.co.uk/2/hi/health/3112170.stm. Accessed 24 Apr 2022.
10. Chung T-T, Lee M-T, Ku M-C, Yang K-C, Wei C-Y. Efficacy of a smart antisnore pillow in patients with obstructive sleep apnea syndrome. Behav Neurol. 2021;2021:8824011. https://doi.org/10.1155/2021/8824011.
11. Zhang J, Zhang Q, Wang Y, Qiu C. A real-time auto-adjustable smart pillow system for sleep apnea detection and treatment. Philadelphia, PA: IEEE; 2013. p. 179–90.
12. Li S, Chiu C. A smart pillow for health sensing system based on temperature and humidity sensors. Sensors. 2018;18(11):3664. https://doi.org/10.3390/s18113664.
13. Zhang Z, Jin X, Wan Z, Zhu M, Wu S. A feasibility study on smart mattresses to improve sleep quality. J Healthc Eng. 2021;2021:6127894. https://doi.org/10.1155/2021/6127894.

Printed by Printforce, the Netherlands